Low Vision

REFLECTIONS OF THE PAST
ISSUES FOR THE FUTURE

Jane N. Erin, Anne L. Corn
and Virginia E. Bishop, editors

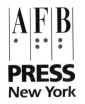

**AFB
PRESS**
New York

Printed in the United States of America

ISBN 0-89128-218-1

The mission of the American Foundation for the Blind (AFB) is to enable persons who are blind or visually impaired to achieve equality of access and opportunity that will ensure freedom of choice in their lives.

CONTENTS

FOREWORD

The symposium and subsequent research survey on which this report is based focused on changes in the field of visual impairment--changes that have taken place in the past 25 years and those that may take place in the years to come. By identifying the shifting needs of people who are visually impaired and the resources that may be needed to address them, *Low Vision: Reflections of the Past, Issues for the Future* examines the realities and trends that have a direct impact on the quality of services for blind and visually impaired people. It is to be hoped that this examination stimulates discussion of how best to provide and improve services. The information contained here can enable administrators to plan and professionals in the field to deliver programs where they are most needed. By improving the quality of services, we by extension improve the quality of life.

Carl R. Augusto
President and Executive Director
American Foundation for the Blind

ACKNOWLEDGMENTS

The authors wish to thank the University of Texas Department of Special Education for its financial and emotional support of this project. The department's farsightedness and commitment to the future of both special education and persons with disabilities have encouraged many important research efforts. The support for the faculty in the Program to Prepare Teachers of the Visually Handicapped is also gratefully appreciated; it is just this kind of encouragement and commitment that allows the teacher preparation program to produce some of the finest special educators in the country.

An additional and very special thanks must go to Dr. James Yates, chair and professor, Department of Educational Administration, the University of Texas at Austin, whose counsel helped add significant meaning to the data reported here. Dr. Yates was a ready adviser on futures methodology and a source of inspiration as well. His belief in the futures approach to research stimulated the ideas incorporated in this project, and his leadership kept it on track.

INTRODUCTION

Many philosophies and practices in the field of education for the visually impaired have turned out to be farsighted and innovative. Public school placements, resource rooms, and itinerant teachers were accepted practices for visually impaired children 20 years before P. L. 94-142 mandated them. Electronic technology was available long before computers and word processing became commonly used. (Magnifying reading systems, such as the Megascope, were developed as early as 1953; obstacle detectors were developed and used in the 1950s and 1960s; computer-generated braille was used in at least one public school system in 1970; and the Optacon emerged in 1971.)

Even the best philosophies and practices have often been accidental, however. Public school placements (and the related itinerant and resource-room service delivery models) occurred because of an unexpected medical phenomenon—retinopathy of prematurity/retrolental fibroplasia. Increased services for deaf-blind children were the result of the rubella epidemic. The development of electronic travel devices resulted primarily from individual efforts, based on the needs of individuals, rather than from farsighted research in the field. Even BrailleEdit grew out of an individual need—a husband's computer expertise applied to meet his wife's needs as a mathematics professor who is blind.

A few innovative ideas for visually impaired persons have even faltered or failed. The IBM braille typewriter seemed like a useful invention at the time, but it never captured the fancy of either blind or sighted users. The large-print edition of the *World Book Encyclopedia* never found its way into school libraries, as had been expected. The Optacon has had limited acceptance by blind users. And many recent electronic devices, both for travel and for communication, are priced so high that they are essentially unavailable to the average visually impaired person.

Clearly, the history of programs and practices in the field of visual impairment has involved much that has been serendipitous and much that has been due to individual initiatives. Professionals—medical, educational, rehabilitation, and technological alike—have reacted more than acted. Instructors in professional preparation programs have been frustrated because their courses involve considerable expertise for low-prevalence needs and cannot, because of the constraints of time, address the full range of skills that are required to work with this ever-changing population.

The solutions to these problems may not be clear or easily identified, but *some* kind of change in philosophy is needed if visually impaired persons are to be adequately prepared for a productive role in society. Considerable foresight is needed to anticipate the long-range needs of today's population of visually impaired people if steps are to be taken now to begin to fulfill them. Moreover, the future needs to be at least somewhat manageable. These qualities—predicting and managing—are what futures research is all about.

Many corporations and governments have been applying futurist techniques for some time. Although each technique approaches forecasting and issues management from a different perspective, all have the same goal: to be prepared for the future.

The project described in this report selected the force-fields analysis approach, since it seemed to have the best possibilities for issues management. Using this approach, researchers collect opinions about future events, examine the probability that these events will occur and their possible impact, and identify the factors that will influence the occurrence of the events. The procedure was first tried at the June 1989 symposium on low vision, "Through the Looking Glass: Reflections of the Past and Visions of the Future," with a captive audience of educators of children with visual impairments, who had come to learn about low vision and to celebrate the 25th anniversary of the Program to Prepare Teachers of the Visually Handicapped at the University of Texas at Austin. The response was so promising that the procedure was utilized in a follow-up study. The present report is both a description of the initial application at the symposium and a detailed account of the follow-up study that was conducted from September to December 1989. Both the papers originally delivered at the symposium and the materials relating to the study are included here. (The papers appear as they were presented, to recapture the symposium's proceedings and to best preserve their original intent.)

The results of both the symposium and the study indicate the need for planned change in the field of visual impairment. It is hoped that readers will take up the challenges and work to realize those benefits that will produce the highest rewards for the visually impaired people of the world.

PART ONE: THE SYMPOSIUM

THROUGH THE LOOKING GLASS

In June 1989, more than 100 graduates of the University of Texas's Program to Prepare Teachers of the Visually Handicapped returned to celebrate the 25th anniversary of the program that prepared them to contribute to the education of visually impaired children. As participants in a field that was in its infancy 25 years ago, these professionals had become advocates for the specialized needs of visually impaired children, both nationally and internationally.

The planning for this celebration had begun more than a year before when two current faculty members, Drs. Anne Corn and Jane Erin, had sought a unique way of celebrating the approaching anniversary of the program. With the administrative skills of Dr. Virginia Bishop, the conference organizer, and the valuable input of Dr. Natalie Barraga, professor emerita and founder of the program, they began to formulate plans for a symposium, to be entitled, "Through the Looking Glass: Reflections of the Past and Visions of the Future." The symposium would examine changes in the field of visual impairment during the program's 25 years and look ahead to the changes that might occur in the next 25 years.

Because a symposium of such national scope would require resources beyond what the program currently maintained, requests for funding to support it were circulated to vendors and professionals in related fields, as well as to a variety of private sources. The College of Education at the university provided substantial financial support and extensive administrative support through its Continuing Education Program. Among the commercial donors were Eschenbach Optik/Duffens Optical; Dickinson Optical; Michael Maki, Optical Design; and Dr. David Starnes, low vision specialist.

The symposium began with a reception at the Arno Nowotny Center, a restored building on the university's campus that was chosen because it had been the original site of the Texas School for the Blind and Visually Impaired. Then called the Blind Asylum, the building opened in 1856 and was staffed by a music teacher and a "literary" teacher. It had been used for the Blind Asylum until 1916, except for a brief period when it served as the headquarters of General George Armstrong Custer during the Civil War. By 1916, when the school was moved to its current site, enrollment had grown to 270 pupils, served by 90 instructors and other staff.

For the evening reception, the period furnishings were complemented by a display of historical educational tools and devices used by visually impaired children (researched and arranged by Dr. Bishop). Included in the display were braillewriters from the turn of the century; examples of tactile reading systems, such as Boston Line type and Moon type; and calculation devices, such as the Taylor slate. Portraits of former superintendents of the Blind Asylum overlooked the display.

At the reception, visitors were welcomed by current and former faculty of the university program, including Drs. Barraga, Corn, Erin, and Bishop. Dr. Waneen Spirduso, interim dean of the College of Education; Dr. J. Lee Wiederholt, chair of the Department of Special Education; and Mr. William Miller, superintendent of the Texas School for the Blind and Visually Impaired, delivered the welcoming remarks. A piano concert was then given by two students from the

Texas School for the Blind, Katsue Tanaka and Masaru Tanaka, under the instruction of Paula Wright.

The following morning, Dr. Barraga began the symposium with a keynote address, "Reflections of the Past." Dr. Barraga transported the audience back to the era when all visually impaired children were educated as if they were blind, regardless of the extent of their useful vision; she recalled the inception of teacher preparation programs in the field and the shift in philosophy toward the importance of encouraging children to use their vision efficiently. Her 1964 study, *Increased Visual Behavior in Low Vision Children,* set the scene for the development of learning options for low vision students; agencies in the field began to address the needs of children who should maximize their use of sight. Dr. Barraga concluded with a challenge to continue the search for knowledge and to use the past to help direct the future.

The participants then heard from four invited speakers who addressed various aspects of the future. Dr. David S. Loshin, of the University of Houston College of Optometry, described innovations in low vision technology, including the Programmable Remapper, which redistributes retinal images so that more information can be viewed by the individual with field defects. A slide and videotape presentation of actual prototypes of this device made theory a reality.

Judith Stotland, a parent and former officer of the National Association for Parents of the Visually Impaired, addressed the future of families of children with visual impairments. She emphasized the changing demographics of families of visually impaired children, stating that in the future, families will be "younger, poorer, and more likely to be from minority cultures." She expressed concern about the ways in which children may be affected by the shortage of specially trained teachers, and underscored the importance of technology and the transdisciplinary team in contributing to the success of the children's education.

Dr. Michael J. Bina, superintendent of the Indiana School for the Blind, spoke about issues related to the future of education of visually impaired students. He shaped his remarks around six Cs: *caring,* in a logical as well as an emotional sense, to send a common message; *conceptualization* of forward-thinking ideas, to address problems within the field; *commitment* to well-defined goals; *collaboration* with those from other fields; *confrontation* of issues that require change; and the *continuation* of efforts to make gains in education.

Finally, Dr. Susan Jay Spungin, associate executive director of the American Foundation for the Blind, addressed futures in the assessment of the learning environment for the student with low vision. She described increasingly rigorous standards and advances in the areas of legislation, medicine, and school-home-community. She described changes in the educational structure, such as the extended school year and the age of mandatory education, that will affect the learning environment, and presented a stimulating menu of possibilities in each of the environments that affect the world of students with low vision. (See Chapters 1–5 for the texts of all the presentations.)

During the afternoon, the participants, under the guidance of Dr. James Yates, chair of the Department of Educational Administration, University of Texas, rated the likelihood and impact of 25 critical future events in the field of visual impairment that had been identified from the morning presentations. After Dr. Yates presented an overview of the forces and strategies related to each event, the participants met in four smaller groups to examine issues in assessment, technology, education, and the family. The groups were moderated by four graduates of the University of Texas's doctoral program in education of visually impaired children: Virginia Bishop, Rita Livingston, Marcia Moore, and Sandy Parsons.

On the basis of the participants' ratings, several critical events were identified, and the four discussion groups utilized force-field analysis to identify the driving forces that may cause an event to happen (facilitators) or prevent it from happening (restrainers). In addition, the Futures Session groups devised strategies to strengthen facilitators in the event of a desirable future event or to strengthen restrainers in the case of an undesirable future event. The remainder of the afternoon was spent in work sessions, in which the participants analyzed their assigned events.

The final activity was a banquet, during which the four group leaders presented the outcomes of their meetings. The audience considered such future possibilities as what may happen if services have not changed by the year 2014 or how education may be affected if more specific contributions were required in the field. (See Chapter 6 for the reports of the session leaders.)

Dr. Barraga then presented "Visions of the Future," in which she described the international activities that provide greater opportunities throughout the world to consider the needs of children with low vision, and she urged the participants to realize their potential to communicate with others on the importance of effective programs and resources. She also challenged them to continue to be active in efforts to serve those with low vision and to become a force for positive change in the future. (See Chapter 7 for Dr. Barraga's remarks.)

Chapter 1

REFLECTIONS OF THE PAST

Dr. Natalie Barraga, Professor Emerita

University of Texas at Austin

Recently, I heard a discussion on memory—the speaker called memory a precious gift, saying that if we can't remember we can't learn. Memory is basic to love, basic to thought, and is important in making us human. Memory is not just our minds or our intelligence but a growing, developing part of our emotional state. Memories are built by acquaintances, relationships, reading, and connecting. We must reinforce our memories if they are to have meaning to us.

In that context, let me suggest that memories and reflections of the past are necessary for us to understand the present, and to visualize the future. "If we don't know where we have been, we have no basis for understanding where we are now, much less a reference for where we might be going in the future."

So turn your mirrors around and look with me at our reflections. For the past 25 years, my professional life has been based right here in Austin at the University of Texas, but I go even further back both personally and professionally in the field of visually handicapped. As a parent, teacher, and subsequently as a teacher-educator, I have 45 years of constant involvement. Let me set the stage by referring to some of the beginnings which are important to our realization of the antiquity of our thinking and behavior in regard to persons with visual impairments. The critical factors relate to changes in philosophy and practices, and seem to center around general attitudes in the field, terminology, organizations and their journals, strategic events, teacher education, and research and literature.

PRIOR TO THE 1940s

In the early years, the entire field of "blindness" was not only influenced, but largely defined by what we know as the medical model in both education and rehabilitation, and by legal requirements and restrictions in terms of eligibility. There was a great dichotomy between the group known as blind according to medical and legal determination, and those called partially seeing by those same standards. All of the former were educated in residential schools along with many of those with low vision, but rarely in the same classrooms or by the same teachers. A few of those with vision were in "sight-saving" classes in local schools as early as 1913. The atmosphere was one of conservation of sight, darkened rooms, and no use of vision lest it disappear. During the 1930s, some of these restrictions were lifted when ophthalmologists began to reverse their previous beliefs of saving sight to suggesting that use of vision did not reduce it nor harm the eyes; however, this applied only to those who were legally defined as "partially seeing" (20/70-20/200), and not to those "legally blind" (20/200 or less) who were actually taught how to be blind.

Residential schools were established by the 1850s and in 1853, the American Instructors of the Blind came into being; by 1872, the name was changed to American Association of Instructors of the Blind (AAIB), and remained so until 1968. This organization was the single most dominant voice in education during those early years when 90 percent of children with visual impairments were educated in residential schools as blind, and only about 10 percent in local schools, the majority of whom had vision.

Many forces were struggling, not always in harmony with each other, so that fractious philosophies were expounded by different people and parts of the country. The *New Outlook for the Blind* was founded by Campbell in 1907, and the National Society for the Prevention of Blindness was organized in 1908 with a distinctly medical focus. They began publishing *Sight-Saving Review* in 1930 and continued until 1985, when it was terminated. The philosophy has always been that of prevention and conservation, and the society continues to function primarily in the areas of screening, prevention, and safety.

After the American Foundation for the Blind (AFB) came into being, they began publication of a *Teacher's Forum* which was absorbed by the *Outlook for the Blind* in 1941. Little communication existed among these groups and organizations—indeed, some tension continued until much later. During these rather tumultuous and unfocused years, there was a rigidity in philosophy and status quo in attitudes and practices. However, when general educational philosophy began to change as a result of research in child development, a few leaders in the field began to see children with visual impairments as individuals belonging to families, rather than objects to be secluded or trained to be robots. Major research was continuing to document that young children thrived and progressed more rapidly when nurtured and cared for by their parents in the early years. This caused some controversial mumblings regarding residential schools, and their appropriateness for all children. The first beginnings of true change in the field of blindness in almost 100 years began to take root.

DECADE OF THE 1940s

There was a decrease in visual impairments in the late 1930s and early 1940s, primarily because of the understanding of genetic causes and a decrease in the numbers of children with hereditary conditions. Also, federal legislation was passed requiring the use of silver nitrate in the eyes of all newborns.

Just when we believed that numbers of children with visual impairments could continue to decrease, along came a new cause. The advent of incubators in hospitals followed by the epidemic of retrolental fibroplasia (RLF) now known as retinopathy of prematurity (ROP) introduced an entirely new population of children. The number of children with visual impairments rose dramatically, and the fact that parents were not inclined or willing to accept the traditional ideas about blindness and the education of children with impairments, caused great changes. There was a 39 percent increase of school-age children with visual impairments from 1949 to 1956. Demands were placed on local schools to provide programs so that children could remain at home, and where teachers and administrators were thought to hold fewer preconceived notions about children with visual impairments.

Summer courses for teachers sprang up in a few areas, some of which were supported by AFB and other organizations. Although Perkins School for the Blind had secured the first university-based program at Harvard (later at Boston University, and subsequently at Boston College), most courses were held only in the summer, with internships at Perkins during the long term. The New York Institute for the Education of the Blind taught courses on their campus with credit given by Hunter College. Summer courses were given also by Teachers College, Columbia University, Peabody College, and Eastern Michigan at Ypsilanti, all of them separate courses for teachers of the "blind," and teachers of the "partially seeing." The vast majority of teachers received only "on-the-job" training at the residential schools. By 1947, the American Printing House for the Blind (APH) began to issue large-print books, and in 1948, the first full-time program in teacher education for visually handicapped began at San Francisco State University with a grant from AFB. Things were rumbling and stirring, but directions were not as yet clear, nor were objectives well defined in any area of the field.

DECADE OF THE 1950s

The decade of the 1950s began with AFB taking a stronger leadership role in teacher education by selecting a full-time person as education specialist, namely Georgia Lee Abel, who went to work immediately by convening national committees to address critical educational issues.

AFB became a clearinghouse for educational ideas, and attempted to "set forth a sane and sympathetic philosophy" for teachers and schools. They defined their role as that of sharing and explaining by publishing the results of the meetings for all to read. Such publications as *Concerning the Education of Blind Children, Itinerant Teaching Service for Blind Children,* and *The Pinebrook Report* are classics, and should be pondered by every prospective and practicing teacher today.

The term *visually handicapped* began to appear as a generic term in the literature, and was used primarily by psychologists and others not a part of the medical/legal/educational "blindness" system. It was much later when it was accepted by organizations and journals in the field, but is still not used universally.

AFB made the services of Miss Abel available during the summers to conduct short courses and/or workshops at colleges and universities upon request. The first course in this field at the University of Texas in Austin was taught by her in 1954, and I had the privilege of attending. From that time, she changed my life both personally and professionally in ways that words have never been able to convey to her. As a low vision person herself, she became the model for this parent of a low vision child, and set my head awhirl with all her innovative and logical ideas about children and their education. Even though she was a product of a residential school herself, and had been a teacher, counselor and principal of one of more, she was one of the strongest advocates of children living at home and attending their local schools whenever possible.

By 1955, APH had established a Division of Research for the sole purpose of defining and studying educational issues, with Dr. Sam Ashcroft as the first director. When he left to coordinate the first full-time program at Peabody College in 1959, Dr. Carson Nolan was appointed. One of his first studies was on the readability of large type, which determined that 18-point type was read more easily than 24- or 36-point type—the first hint that bigger may not be better for all vision students. The use of optical aids for low vision persons was being experimented with, but almost exclusively with adults. New ideas began to emerge, but still there was little consensus or focus in educational programming.

THE PROGRESSIVE 1960s

A virtual explosion of ideas and knowledge started coming together in the decade of the 1960s despite the negative factors beginning to change the society around us. The Council for Exceptional Children was having an impact on the U.S. Office of Education, and upon teachers in the local schools who formed the Division of Visually Handicapped. This action flamed the controversy of residential schools versus public schools, and for a time, a great chasm seemed to divide educators and inhibit communication and singleness of purpose.

About this time, the Mental Retardation Act had been passed, and there was leadership at the Federal level for all aspects of education including special education. A Bureau for Education for the Handicapped (BEH) was formed, and Jack Jones was appointed as a specialist in visually handicapped. He immediately began to conduct surveys and studies to determine the "state of the art." A very significant survey was that of print and braille readers in residential and public schools related to their degrees of vision. A startling 50 percent of low vision children in public schools read print, whereas only 29 percent of those in residential settings were print readers. Some residential schools were still covering children's hands, putting paper sacks over their heads, or blindfolding children with vision to prevent them reading braille with the eyes. A leading ophthalmologist, Dr. Gerald Fonda, published a guide to the use of optical aids, and declared "it is a disservice to teach a person braille when he/she could read print as fast or faster with an optical aid."

Meanwhile, administrators at the University of Texas were thinking ahead also. After the passage of the Mental Retardation Act, they knew that it would just be a matter of time before that was extended to other handicapping conditions. So in 1960, the finger was pointed to me. After I completed my master's in 1957, I had been conducting a demonstration class, and teaching courses during the summer, so I was challenged to "go away and complete your doctorate, and come back on our faculty full time." Much to their surprise, probably, and indeed to mine, I said, "Why not? I need a new challenge after teaching at residential schools for more than 10 years." Did I ever get a challenge!

By the time I arrived at Peabody College in 1961 to study and work with Dr. Ashcroft, I had no idea that the world of literature and learning was so rich and wide open to me, and that there was so much to know. But sadly, I soon came to realize that even though we knew so much, we were only putting into practice a small fraction of that knowledge to help change the lives of visually handicapped children and youth (which I am sorry to say is still true today to some extent).

Although the discrepancy I had been experiencing between children called "blind" and their functional behavior had bothered me for years, I hadn't known what to do about it. Somehow I couldn't find the right questions to ask in order to try to find some answers. Then in 1961, Barbara Bateman completed her dissertation at the University of Illinois entitled *Reading and Psycholinguistic Processes of Partially Seeing Children,* in which she came to the following conclusions:

> "If the suggestion from this study that central processes are not necessarily grossly impaired by limitations on sensory input is sound, the implications are profound. Even though the end organ may be defective and grossly limit the sensations received centrally, the central processes can perhaps "set-up" the magnitude of stimulation or accuracy of perception. Theoretical justification has been presented for continuing with increased zeal an already established precept in special education—helping each child to use centrally what he has peripherally."

Lights flashed, bells rang, my heart beat wildly, and my brain seemed to explode. "We've been concerned about what the eyes could *not* do, when we should have been worrying about what the brain *can* do." Trying to put it all together, I buried myself in the library with medical, psychological, optometric, neurological, child development, and educational literature until a theoretical basis for a study could be formulated. This theory had to make sense from a developmental and learning point of view, be compatible with research in other disciplines, and incidentally pass the scrutiny of my committee.

In 1963, the first scientific study documenting that use of vision and visual efficiency were learned processes and could be taught established the fact that low vision was not a static entity in the eye nor related solely to acuity measurement, but was indeed amenable to change in learning and functional behavior. About this time, the *Outlook for the Blind* published an article by Barnes, who advocated that the term *sight utilization* replace the terms *sight-saving* and *sight conservation*. Mr. Lee Sanborn, a well-respected residential school superintendent, wrote an article on the use of optical aids by low vision children in his school. It was comforting to know that others were beginning to promote similar ideas.

As soon as AFB published *Increased Visual Behavior in Low Vision Children* in 1964, Pandora's box seemed to open. Was this a fluke? Could we really teach children how to use their vision more efficiently? Maybe my intense desire, unique teaching style, or the special materials I made were the key rather than the principle and the process. The ultimate test was for the study to be replicated with different teachers, different children, and materials available in the schools but following the process and the same sequence of lessons. Ashcroft and Halliday completed their study in 1965, followed by a similar study with older youth by Holmes in 1967. By then, the pot was simmering all over the country, but being doused regularly by skeptics who were not ready to give up traditional ideas and methods.

Katie Sibert in California wrote an article about "the legally blind child with useful vision," substantiating her work with children in a public school resource room. Dr. Fonda published an article, "Evaluation of Large Type," and concluded with this question, "Why rely on large type when one can read regular type with or without aids?" Dr. Nolan was conducting studies consistently on the reading media of students registered with APH. In 1966, 46 percent of legally blind students still used braille, but this had dropped to 39 percent by 1969. However, even students with higher degrees of vision continued to use braille in residential schools. The first presentations on low vision and optical aids were made at the AAIB convention in 1968. Gradual awakening and acceptance were coming slowly. AAIB even changed the name of the organization to Educators of the Visually Handicapped (EVH) and the name of the IJEB [*International Journal for the Education of the Blind*] to EVH in 1968, but not without strong opposition.

When I returned to the University of Texas as an assistant professor in 1963, just as the dean had predicted, federal funds were made available for teacher education for all disabling conditions. Our proposal was one of the first submitted, and the first funding began in the 1964-65 school year. The program has received continuous funding for these 25 years including the present. Programs around the nation grew from two (San Francisco State and Peabody College) to 27 full-time programs in 17 different states by 1972. Not all programs included all levels of undergraduate, master's, and doctoral, and a few had courses at only one or the other of these levels.

The University of Texas has given full administrative and professional support for this program from the beginning, using the federal funds for start-up of faculty salaries, with gradual assumption of state support, so that faculty have all been on "hard money" for several years. Federal funds have been used for stipends for students, expensive equipment, research assistants, and for travel and other enrichment activities and materials. Without the university's recognition of the need for this program, and their full support, we could not be here today celebrating our survival when so many programs are folding elsewhere.

The establishment of the program here deviated from some of the more traditional standards previously set. For example, this was the first program to offer one set of courses to prepare teachers to work with all visually handicapped children, with no separate tracks for blind and partially seeing; in fact, those terms have never appeared in any course title. This program was also the first to use both an ophthalmologist and an optometrist as clinical consultants to a visual problems course taught by an educator who could emphasize the educational implications of visual etiologies for the classroom teacher. Most programs had a medical person teach an "eye" course or it may even have been taught by someone in the biology department, and some even follow this pattern today.

Perhaps the program took a step away from the "medical" model to the "educational model" by the philosophy, course names, and in providing information about the options available in placement and media preference—decisions to be made jointly by parents and teachers, rather than dictated by a medical person.

The bomb fell and the dam broke in 1969, when Dr. James Moss, director of the Division of Research, BEH, startled me and everyone else in a presentation at the annual meetings at APH. He challenged residential school superintendents, trustees of state departments of

11

education, and teacher-educators to use the low vision studies as a model from which research findings could be disseminated to classroom teachers. By the close of 1969, under the leadership of Jo Taylor (who had replaced Jack Jones as vision specialist at BEH), a committee of national leaders in visually handicapped had met in Austin to develop a plan of action for emphasizing the utilization of low vision with every child. This group left having established a cooperative agreement between BEH, APH, and the colleges and universities in a nationwide effort to translate research findings into classrooms for visually handicapped.

ACTION IN THE 1970s

Needless to say, the 1970s began with a bang and long overdue progress became the concern of the entire field. A number of events, books, articles, and research have characterized the last two decades. It all began with a series of 15 Low Vision Institutes, funded by BEH, sponsored by colleges and universities with materials furnished and disseminated by APH to more than 500 participants all over the United States from 1970 to 1972. Teachers themselves were getting the message, and things were beginning to happen for low vision children and youth.

Research on print reading by visually handicapped was done by Dr. Kim Sykes in 1971-72. He found that high school students, when provided with magnifying devices from which to choose, and special lamps or lighting arrangements, were just as efficient with regular-sized print as they were with large-print materials; some of them with lower degrees of vision were more efficient with regular-size type; reading regular-size print was no more tiring than large print. (We seem not to have put this into practice even yet.)

Dr. Michael Tobin, in England, conducted a study similar to the 1963 low vision study with children registered as "legally blind" in schools for the blind in that country. He found the same results as we had, and provided further evidence of the nature of vision as a perceptual/cognitive process, rather than a phenomenon related to sight.

There was still very little literature from which to draw, but *The Visually Handicapped Child* by Bishop in 1971 was welcomed by teachers in public schools especially, followed by the book edited by Dr. Berthold Lowenfeld, *The Visually Handicapped Child in School,* written by ten of us and published by AFB. A book by Dr. Eleanor Faye (an ophthalmologist) and Clare Hood at the Low Vision Clinic of the New York Lighthouse for the Blind was published in 1975; later, in 1976, Dr. Faye came out with *Clinical Low Vision,* directed to both ophthalmologists and optometrists.

Dr. Ozias, one of the doctoral graduates of the University of Texas, completed his study of the effectiveness of special study institutes as dissemination vehicles. He found that after the first 15 institutes in 1970-71, 47 others had been conducted by many of those first participants. Thousands of teachers were getting information about low vision and the teaching of visual efficiency in functional use. He also elicited and received suggestions from teachers for improvement of the *Visual Efficiency Scale* and the teaching materials disseminated in those institutes. If you don't want teachers of visually handicapped to tell you what they want and need, don't ask them. We spent a year collating all their suggestions, and deciding how to meet some of those desires in the future. Their responses were invaluable in our subsequent research and development project.

Dr. Carson Nolan at APH agreed that we needed a revision of the low vision materials, so with our collaboration, a 3-year research and development proposal was submitted and funded by the U.S. Office of Education. The objectives were to revise assessment procedures, develop definitive instructional lessons and materials, field test both of these, and provide a book on low vision. A national advisory committee included members from every element of the field and from every related discipline, to work in concert with a team from APH and a team from the University of Texas at Austin, a time many of us will never forget.

While this work was proceeding, other events and publications were continuing. AFB appointed a low vision advisory committee, which resulted in the appointment of a low vision consultant to the AFB staff. A manual for teachers, *Vision Stimulation,* was developed and published by Montgomery County, Maryland, under the direction of Rosemary O'Brien. Some colleges and universities conducted their own institutes, and Illinois State University published their proceedings. Slowly but surely, the word was gradually being heard, and more and more people were believing. Parents became involved, and wanted to help their preschool children especially. In Canada, Eileen Scott published a book for parents, *Can't Your Child See?* which was read by parents in the United States and elsewhere.

A NEW ERA BEGINS

The highlight of the 1980s began with the arrival of Dr. Anne Corn to join our faculty in visually handicapped. We had searched long and hard for just the right person, and I know that you will agree with me that we found her. Dr. Corn had lived what I have only observed and theorized about, and she continues to bring new insights about functional low vision to me and others every day. Her studies on optical aids and her theoretical model for individuals with low vision are evidence of a bright future. You as alumni and the University of Texas can expect great things from this program in the next 25 years as Dr. Corn and Dr. Jane Erin continue to make beautiful music.

Other studies in low vision have been completed by Dr. Sandy Parsons, now at the University of South Carolina, and Dr. Rita Livingston at the Pennsylvania College of Optometry, along with a few from other institutions. It is only the beginning—there is still so much we need to investigate.

A factor which has had a great impact on our reflections and challenged us to even greater lengths began in 1963 with a rubella epidemic. Thousands of children were impaired both visually and auditorally, many of whom were later found to have neurological and cognitive damage as well. Technology has brought us many tools, but it has also brought us headaches. The changing society, relaxation of some standards, altered values, and even some hedonistic tendencies, are a part of the new challenges to the medical and educational communities which have yet to be resolved. Retinopathy of prematurity (ROP), once thought a thing of the past, is again with us. Along with tools for efficiency in functioning, advanced technology has given us children who 15 years ago would not have survived, but today need our services. These children may be an even greater enigma to teachers than were low vision children in the '50s and '60s.

The entire population of multihandicapped children and knowledge of how best to serve them is one of your problems for the future. Because we have barely scratched the surface in understanding their needs, much less their capabilities and real limitations, there is much research and creative thinking needed in the next decade. Pennsylvania College of Optometry published *Look at Me,* which is a good beginning for teachers to get ideas for objectives and tasks to be used with this group. Dr. Erin had valuable experience with this group, and along with Dr. Corn, this program may be the key to a new breakthrough in the next 25 years.

Apparently a great impact has been made in low vision with the 1980 publication by APH of *Program to Develop Efficiency in Visually Functioning,* both in this country and around the world. To my knowledge, it has been translated into at least 6 additional languages for use of teachers in non-English speaking countries. Would you believe that I have visited two schools in the United States in the last two months who have not yet heard of or made use of those materials? Maybe we haven't come as far as we think!

The establishment of a clinical/educational program to train vision specialists at the master's level at Pennsylvania College of Optometry is beginning to fill a need and foster interdisciplinary communication as teachers, mobility instructors, and clinicians work together and focus on low vision and use of optical aids. This program promises to have an even greater future by the addition of an educator of the staff as Dr. Rita Livingston becomes associate director for continuing education and international programs.

Understanding Low Vision, by Dr. Randy Jose, published by AFB in 1983, is now widely used in low vision clinics, colleges and universities, and has also been translated into Spanish.

As we look to the future, which you will spend the next day doing, please realize that YOU ARE THE FUTURE. Your commitment, your dedication, and your intensity will be reflected in your day work with children and youth, but more importantly in your leadership and research. You will be asking the right questions, seeking better answers, pushing for legislation, and never being satisfied with the status quo. Your loyalty to this program will help to keep it strong and innovative.

We have awakened, but I am not sure we have the scales from our eyes as yet. There is much to do, and I know that you, as great alumni and students of this program, along with your capable leaders, Dr. Corn and Dr. Erin, with the continued support of this grand university will make a positive impact in the next 25 years. Thanks for all the cherished memories.

REFERENCES

Abel, G. L. (Ed.). (1959). *Concerning the education of blind children.* New York: American Foundation for the Blind.

American Foundation for the Blind. (1954). *The Pinebrook report: National work session on the education of the blind with the sighted.* New York: Author.

American Foundation for the Blind. (1957). *Itinerant teaching service for blind children.* New York: Author.

Ashcroft, S. C., Halliday, C., & Barraga, N. C. (1965). *Study II: Effects of experimental teaching on the visual behavior of children educated as though they had no vision.* Nashville, TN: George Peabody College, Vanderbilt University.

Barraga, N. C. (1964). *Increased visual behavior in low vision children.* New York: American Foundation for the Blind.

Barraga, N. C. (1970). *Visual Efficiency Scale.* Louisville, KY: American Printing House for the Blind.

Barraga, N. C., & Morris, J. (1980). *Program to develop efficiency in visual functioning.* Louisville, KY: American Printing House for the Blind.

Barnes, F. J. (1963). Let's call it "sight utilization." *New Outlook for the Blind, 57,* 97-98.

Bateman, B. (1963). *Reading and psycholinguistic processes of partially seeing children* (CEC Monograph, Series A, No. 5). Arlington, VA.: Council for Exceptional Children.

Bishop, V. (1971). *Teaching the visually limited child.* Springfield, IL: Charles C Thomas.

Corn, A. (1981). Optical aids in the classroom. *Education of the Visually Handicapped, 12,* 114-121.

Corn, A. (1983). Visual function: A model for individuals with low vision. *Journal of Visual Impairment & Blindness, 77,* 373-377.

Faye, E. E. (1976). *Clinical low vision.* Boston: Little, Brown.

Faye, E. E., & Hood, C. M. (Eds.). (1975). *Low vision.* Springfield, IL: Charles C Thomas.

Fonda, G. (1965). *Management of the patient with subnormal vision.* St. Louis, MO: C. V. Mosby.

Fonda, G. (1966). An evaluation for large type. *New Outlook for the Blind, 60,* 296-298.

Holmes, R. B. (1967). *Training residual vision in adolescents educated previously as nonvisual.* Unpublished master's degree thesis, Illinois State University, Normal.

Jose, R. (1983). *Understanding low vision.* New York: American Foundation for the Blind.

Kederis, C., & Ashcroft, S. C. (1970). The Austin conference on utilization of low vision. *Education of the Visually Handicapped, 2,* 33–38.

Livingston, R. K. (1984). *Abilities of students with low vision to quickly identify projected outline drawings of familiar objects from distances of 6 and 10 feet.* Unpublished doctoral dissertation, University of Texas at Austin.

Lowenfeld, B. (Ed.). (1973). *The visually handicapped child in school.* New York: John Day.

Nolan, C. Y. (1959). Readability of large type: A study of type sizes and type styles. *International Journal for the Education of the Blind, 9,* 41–44.

O'Brien, R. (Ed.). (1971). *Vision stimulation.* (Bulletin 227). Rockville, MD: Montgomery County Public Schools.

Ozias, D. K. (1975). *An evaluation of a research information dissemination and translation vehicle: Special study institutes on utilization of low vision.* Unpublished doctoral dissertation, the University of Texas at Austin.

Parsons, A. A. (1982). *An exploratory study on the patterns of emerging play behavior in young children with low vision.* Unpublished doctoral dissertation, University of Texas at Austin.

Rex, E. (Ed.). (1971). *Proceedings of a special study institute: Methods and procedures for training low vision skills.* Normal: Illinois State University.

Sanborn, L. C. (1963). The partially sighted child in a school for the blind. *New Outlook for the Blind, 57,* 191–194.

Scott, E. P., (1977). *Can't your child see?* Baltimore, MD.: University Park Press.

Sibert, K. N. (1966). The legally blind child with useful residual vision. *International Journal for the Education of the Blind, 16,* 33–44.

Smith, A. J., & Cote, K. S. (1982). *Look at me.* Philadelphia: Pennsylvania College of Optometry Press.

Sykes, K. C. (1971). A comparison of the effectiveness of standard print in facilitating the reading skills of visually impaired students. *Education of the Visually Handicapped, 3,* 97–105.

Sykes, K. C. (1972). Print reading for visually handicapped children. *Education of the Visually Handicapped, 4,* 71–75.

Tobin, M. J. (1973). *A study in the improvement of visual efficiency in children registered as blind.* Birmingham, England: University of Birmingham Research Center for the Education of the Visually Handicapped.

Chapter 2

FUTURES IN TECHNOLOGY

David S. Loshin, O.D., Ph.D.

University of Houston

As low vision professionals, we are currently limited as to what we can actually do for our patients. Teaching the patient how to cope with the visual problem is a large part of the rehabilitative process. Many times, trivial alterations in how a patient performs a task can lead to major improvement. For example, individuals with cataracts or age-related maculopathy (ARM) can read much more effectively if the lighting is properly adjusted. Currently, the bulk of coping aids are optical devices which magnify. Hand-held and stand magnifiers, telescopes, microscopes, closed-circuit televisions (CCTVs) all have uniform magnification throughout and thus increase the scale of the image which falls on the patient's retina. For the patient who has a central field defect, a portion of the retinal image, which would otherwise normally fall within the defect, is extended onto viable peripheral retina. This permits the patient to regain at least part of the lost central field information; however, it is at the expense of losing a portion of the peripheral field. For low magnifications and certain tasks, this may not cause a problem. For higher magnifications, the resulting reduced field size restricts the amount of the world that may be seen at one time and the patient must integrate the partial views into a whole image. This is extremely difficult for certain tasks such as facial recognition, where a glimpse of the eyes, hair, forehead, nose, etc. is arduous to integrate into a perception of a face that can be identified.

When the field defect involves the peripheral retina, as in cases of retinitis pigmentosa (RP), a different type of visual problem results. This restricted peripheral field can lead to tunnel vision, which makes mobility difficult. Here, a reverse telescope may be prescribed. This device uniformly minifies the retinal image so that peripheral field information falls onto viable central retina. The reverse telescope is somewhat effective as long as the acuity of the central retina is capable of resolving sufficient detail in the reduced image.

When one is viewing through these optical devices, spatial localization of objects within the field is often compromised. Therefore, the devices are rarely used for constant viewing. Patients usually alternate between viewing the field directly and spotting objects through the aid. Typically, low vision aids are not used when the patient is walking, since head and body motion amplifies the movement of the resulting retinal image, making it even more difficult to interpret.

New technology in electro-optics has stimulated development of a new generation of low vision devices. Future reductions in cost and size along with added versatility may permit aids to be "programmed" according to individual patient requirements for a specific pathology or task. One such proposed low vision device is a spectacle-mounted display unit (Figure 1).
A head-mounted, miniaturized television camera will provide the image of the world. Since the location of the field defect relative to the fixation should remain constant, feedback indicating

the eye position may be required. If the camera's optics are carried on their head (perhaps using an unobtrusive fiber optic link), patients may also be trained to move their head for a new view and simply fixate the center of the display image. A considerable reduction in system complexity results. A display system somewhat similar to this exists as prototype at both NASA [National Aeronautics and Space Administration] (Ames and JSC [Johnson Space Center]) for applications on the space station.

The display unit is not the only future low vision advancement. Images displayed through this unit may be enhanced so that they may be more easily seen by the low vision patient. I will discuss two such techniques for enhancement currently being explored. One technique involves enhancement of the contrast through electronic filtering. I will discuss these techniques briefly. The other enhancement technique is called image remapping. I will present this technique in some detail, since I have been intimately involved in its development. [*Note:* Figures 7, 8, 10, and 11, which were part of this original presentation, were shown as slides. They therefore do not appear in this volume. For information about these figures, readers should contact the author.]

CONTRAST ENHANCEMENT

In vision testing, we routinely measure visual acuity, i.e., the smallest, high-contrast letter one can recognize. From this measurement, an index of how well someone sees is established. We assume an individual with 20/20 acuity sees well and one with 20/400 acuity sees poorly. Unfortunately, visual acuity is a poor predictor of how well we perform daily living tasks. In everyday life we are faced with detection and recognition of many objects with various sizes and contrast levels. In order to assess visual performance more thoroughly, the contrast level required for detection over a range of object sizes encountered in daily living should be determined. This is accomplished through contrast sensitivity testing. Contrast sensitivity testing may be compared to auditory testing, where the amplitude (volume) for detection of different tones or temporal frequencies is determined.

There are several methods used to measure contrast sensitivity. In all cases, the visual stimulus is either gratings with a sinusoidal luminance profile or letters. In our laboratory apparatus, a sinusoidual grating is presented on an oscilloscope screen at a suprathreshold level and reduced in contrast until it disappears. After a brief delay, the disappearance and reappearance of the grating by pushing a button interfaced with a computer. The contrast level is plotted on the computer monitor as data is being collected, which allows for retesting of questionable values. This process is repeated with several gratings with different spatial frequencies.

As shown in Figure 2, this contrast data is plotted as long contrast sensitivity (ordinate) versus log spatial frequency (abscissa). The resulting curve is called the contrast sensitivity function or CSF. The normal CSF has a characteristic bell shape with a peak at approximately 4 to 6 c/deg. There is a fall-off for frequencies below the peak due to the neural mechanisms of the eye. Note that this means that larger objects may require more contrast than objects that are of moderate size. For frequencies above the peak, more and more contrast is required as the grating gets smaller (higher frequencies). The intersection of the curve with the x-axis represents the high frequency cut-off or resolution acuity. This point may be compared to the letter acuity described. In the normal CSF in Figure 2, the resolution acuity is approximately 40 c/deg, which represents a letter acuity of 20/15. It should be clear that letter acuity yields only one point in the spatial frequency spectrum.

In visual pathology, the CSF is usually altered; the curve is lowered and shifted toward lower spatial frequencies (Fig. 2). Deficient spatial frequencies may be identified and selectively enhanced. This is the basis for contrast enhancement. It should be noted that enhancement may not have the same requirements for all tasks, i.e., different tasks may be different critical frequencies that required enhancement. Recent experimentation with contrast enhancement has been performed with reading and facial recognition.

Lawton (1988) has reported a contrast enhancement technique by electronically filtering printed material based upon the individual patient's CSF. This process is performed at video rates using an electronic chip developed at NASA JPL. Lawton has tested the effectiveness of the technique by measuring reading rate of patients with age-related maculopathy. Although experimentation is ongoing, preliminary results show as much as 4x reading rate increase with filtered images. This is mainly due to the fact that less magnification is required with filtered letters.

Many patients with age-related maculopathy (ARM) have difficulty in recognizing faces. Loshin and Banton (1988) have reported that the contrast of the lower face is critical in the discrimination of faces for patients with ARM. Several investigators have shown different techniques for contrast filtering which may enhance facial recognition (Schuchard & Rubin, 1989; Goldstein & Peli, 1989). From these preliminary experiments, contrast enhancement appears to increase the ability to recognize faces.

Contrast enhancement will be one technique which will be incorporated in future low vision devices.

IMAGE REMAPPING

We have been experimenting with the potential of a device called the Programmable Remapper as a low vision aid. The Programmable Remapper, which is a digital-image processor of unique design and function, has been developed at NASA, Johnson Space Center. The remapper was designed to perform coordinate transformations in real-time on video images. Other digital-image processors, for the most part, perform point operations on an image; that is, the pixel values are changed, but the shapes and locations of objects within the field are not disturbed. The remapper, on the other hand, can change spatial relationships as well as the position of objects within the field by reassigning the location for each pixel. This image warping is controlled by algorithms developed for specific operations. The original intent of the remapper was to simplify some aspects of pattern recognition in video imagery. NASA's interest arises from problems in automated tracking and docking of spacecraft and in autonomous landings on Mars.

The remapper's potential application to human low vision became apparent early in its development. In diseases which result in obvious field defects such as age-related maculopathy (ARM) or retinitis pigmentosa (RP), the remapper can be used to redistribute, onto still-viable retina, image information that would otherwise be lost due to the field defect. Not only can the remapper emulate the uniform minification or magnification of the current low vision devices, but it can also perform unique coordinate transformations. Thus the constraints dictated by optics can be lifted and improvements in the design of a low vision prosthesis could be possible.

We envision the remapper as a fundamental component of a low vision prosthesis. The remapper, carried as a portable unit, will warp the image in a manner customized for the individual user. To date, however, we have not concentrated on the exact requirements of this low vision system, but rather, on the potential of video-rate, low lag-image warping as a low vision aid. If other military, space and/or industrial applications for the remapper provide the economic motivation, the system could be reduced to a multi-purpose, VLSI wafer scale unit.

We have developed preliminary algorithms for remapping images for patients with central or peripheral field defects. In this presentation, we will present the process of image remapping under these conditions as well as examples of remapped static images. In many cases, this process results in image distortion; however, initial experimentation has indicated that this distortion may be acceptable if accompanied by significant visual improvement. Distortion is a trade-off against amount of information available to the brain for interpretation. Previous experiments have shown that with optically induced distortion with inverting, displacing, and reversing prisms (Cohen, 1965; Cranshaw & Craske, 1974; Droules & Cornilleau, 1987; Hay & Pick, 1966; Kohler, 1962), both visumotor and perceptual adaptation is possible. In addition, one must remember that the remapper presents dynamic images, not static ones. This will not only permit changes in the amount of distortion (as controlled by the patient) but also allow alternation between several views (remapped and not remapped) of the visual world.

In the work we have completed, we used the remapper to alter the eccentricities of pixels in an image. Figure 3 shows some of the relation between eccentricity measured in the world (i.e., relative to the input camera's optical axis) and eccentricity presented to the eye (i.e., in the display of the warped image). The abscissa is world eccentricity, the ordinate is retinal eccentricity. The axes have been arbitrarily partitioned into central and peripheral regions. Status of the fields is indicated in the shaded regions beside the abscissa and ordinate. The 45 degree line in Figure 3 represents a null warping; input and output eccentricities are the same, and all points in the viewed world appear in their normal locations.

Figure 4 shows this diagram for a central field defect. The retinal axis is labeled with the defect. The information in the world field corresponding to this retinal field falls within the defect and therefore is lost, while the peripheral field remains the same as in the normal condition. With optical magnification, the relationship between the spatial and retinal fields is altered. This is shown in Figure 5 by a new transfer line having a different slope. Part of the information that would be lost within the field defect is magnified beyond the extreme of the retinal field. This results in the reduced field of view produced by most magnifying optical aids.

The algorithm we developed to remap images for central field defects yields a transfer line indicated in Figure 6. The central portion of the spatial field is remapped onto the retinal position at the edge of the field defect. The extreme peripheral spatial field is remapped onto the extreme peripheral retinal field. All other spatial positions are remapped onto the retinal field between these positions and thus the entire spatial field falls within the viable retina. This type of remapping yields what we call a zero effective scotoma.

Figure 7 displays grids that have undergone this process. [*Note:* Figures 7, 8, 10, and 11 do not accompany the present text, as explained earlier.] In the upper left of Figure 7, a grid in the spatial field obscured by a scotoma is shown without remapping. The information falling within the defect is lost. The grids that have undergone uniform magnification and zero effective scotoma remappings are shown in the upper right and lower left, respectively. With the uniform magnification and zero effective scotoma remappings are shown in the upper right and lower left, respectively. With the uniform magnification, the number of zones in the grid are reduced, indicating a reduction in the field of view. The zero effective scotoma has distortion. The remapping, however, is obvious if you follow the central vertical and horizontal lines to and around the field defect.

The same remapping algorithm has been applied to printed material in Figure 8 (no remapping left and remapped image right). The image represents approximately a 3x7 scotoma at 40cm. The words that would fall within the defect are "stretched" above, below, and to the left and right of the defect. An added enhancement of this process is the magnification of the letters at the edge of the field defect. With a modification in the algorithm, reading material could be packed to the left of fixation, which may help individuals who lose their place on the line while reading. The actual remapping process is dynamic; the remapped field could follow the position of the eye if required.

As shown in Figure 9, peripheral field defects can be diagrammed using the same scheme we used to display the central field defects. The information from the peripheral spatial field will fall within the peripheral retinal field defect using the 45 transfer line. The conventional reverse telescopic aid will uniformly minify, which can be shown using the transfer line as indicated. All the information within the spatial field is reduced in size so that it can fall onto viable retina. An alternative method, as shown in Figure 8, is to remap the central field with a curve near the 45 line gradually approaching the edge of the field defect with a curved transfer line. This remapping allows a choice among a parameterized family of curves. As the curve parameter increases, more of the central field remains unchanged and the noncentral image is squeezed at the edge of the viable retina. This results in a programmable "fish-eye lens" effect.

For a particular family of curves (Loshin & Juday, 1989) with a single continuously variable parameter, Figure 10 displays this remapping process on the grid for several different parameter values. The grid in the upper left of Figure 9 represents a reduced field. A parameter of unity uniformly minifies and thus acts as a standard reverse telescope correction (Figure 10, upper right). As the factor is increased, the grid in the central field approaches the unremapped grid size (Figure 10, lower left and right). In Figure 11, a scene is shown with a reduced field (upper left), with uniform minification (upper right), and after being remapped with two different values of the parameter (lower left and right). If an individual intended to walk to the dark oven in the center of the scene, the unremapped field will not yield enough information; however, spatial localization in the field is severely degraded. With the proper remapping factor, the central oven can be displayed at approximately full size, while the peripheral field, although distorted, can provide adequate information about the field to allow safe mobility. Since the remapper is dynamic and in its present form has the capability to store several different remapping tables, the output scene could be stepped through several parameter values, allowing the patient to select one that best suits the situation.

These preliminary studies do not controvert the validity of remapping as an improved form of low vision aid. Low vision patients who have been shown the static remapped print have indicated that the print is "easier" to see. This system will provide dynamic remapping (which will be shown as a video tape in the presentation). The present system will use an input-output similar to a CCTV. The patient will look at the center of the screen and the text will be moved on the reading table under the camera. An eye monitor will be added to the system when it becomes available. We hope to report on this clinical investigation in the near future.

Figure 1

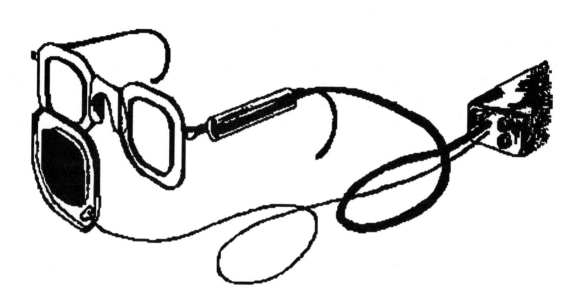

Figure 2

CONTRAST SENSITIVITY FUNCTIONS

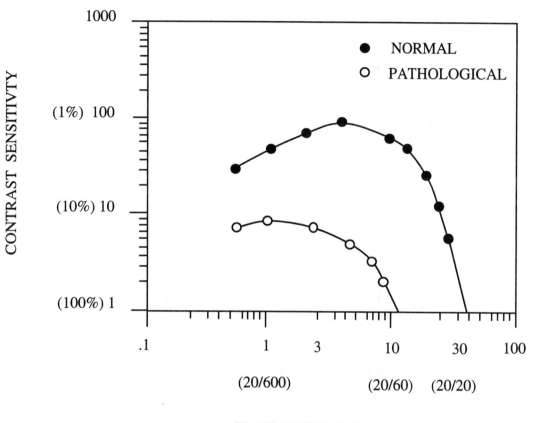

SPATIAL FREQUENCY (c/deg)

Figure 3

DIAGRAMMATIC REPRESENTATION OF MAPPING
THE VISUAL FIELD ONTO THE RETINA

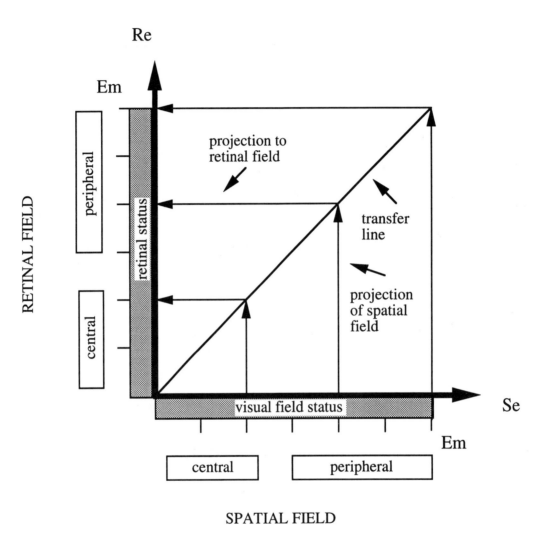

SPATIAL FIELD

Em = Maximum eccentricity
Re = Retinal eccentricity
Se = Spatial eccentricity

Figure 4

CENTRAL FIELD DEFECT
NO REMAPPING

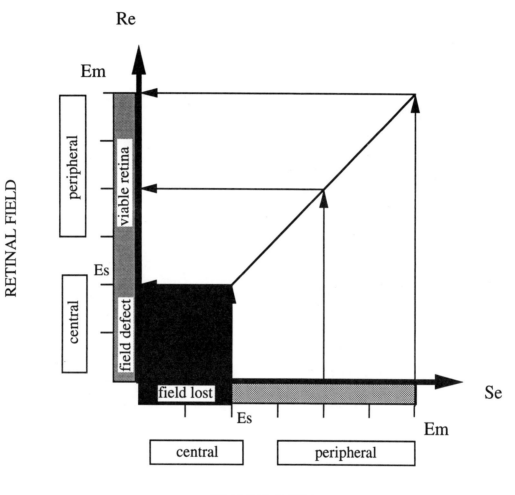

Em = Maximum eccentricity
Re = Retinal eccentricity
Se = Spatial eccentricity
Es = Scotoma eccentricity

Figure 5

CENTRAL FIELD DEFECT
UNIFORM MAGNIFICATION

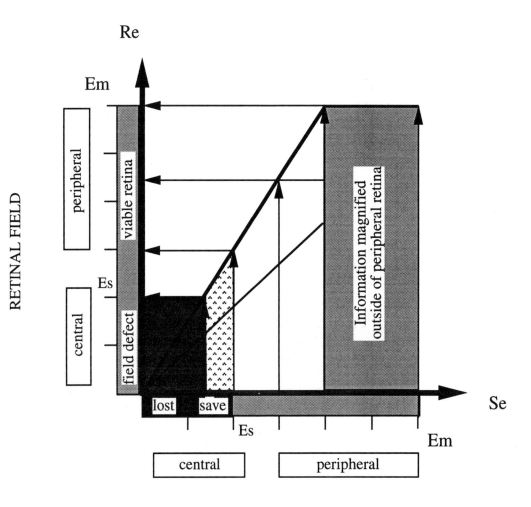

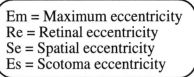

Em = Maximum eccentricity
Re = Retinal eccentricity
Se = Spatial eccentricity
Es = Scotoma eccentricity

Figure 6

CENTRAL FIELD DEFECT
ZERO EFFECTIVE SCOTOMA

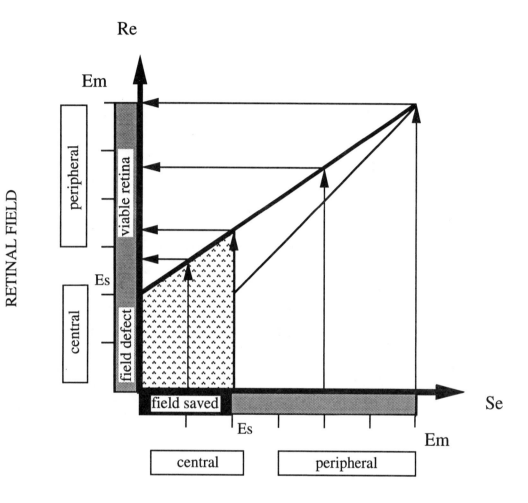

Em = Maximum eccentricity
Re = Retinal eccentricity
Se = Spatial eccentricity
Es = Scotoma eccentricity

Figure 9

PERIPHERAL FIELD DEFECT
REPRESENTATIVE REMAPPING

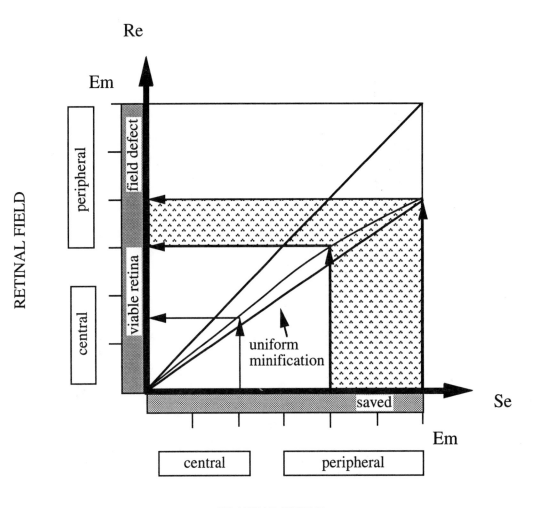

Em = Maximum eccentricity
Re = Retinal eccentricity
Se = Spatial eccentricity
Es = Scotoma eccentricity

REFERENCES

Cohen, H. B. (1965). Some critical factors in prism adaptation. *American Journal of Psychology, 79,* 285-290.

Cranshaw, M., & Craske, B. (1974). No retinal component in prism adaptation. *Acta Psychologica, 38,* 421-423.

Droules, J., & Cornilleau, V. (1987). Adaptive changes in perception responses and visuomanual coordination during exposure to metrical distortion. *Vision Research, 26,* 1783-1792.

Fisher, T. E., & Juday, R. D. (1988). A programmable image remapper. *SPIE Vol. 938, Digital and Optical Shape Representation and Pattern Recognition,* 122-128.

Goldstein, R., & Peli, E. (1989). Simulation of low-vision perception of images and the CSF. *Investigative Ophthalmology and Visual Science (supplement) 30,* 397.

Hay, J. C., & Pick, H. L. (1966). Visual and proprioceptive adaptation to optical displacement of the visual stimulus. *Journal of Experimental Psychology, 71,* 150-158.

Kohler, I. (1964). The formation of the perceptual world. *Psychological Issues, 3* (Monograph 12), 5-166.

Lawton, T. (1988). Improved word recognition for observers with age-related maculopathies using compensation filters. *Clinical Vision Sciences, 3,* 125-135.

Loshin, D. S., & Banton, T. (1988). Local contrast requirements for facial recognition in patients with central field defects. *Investigative Ophthalmology and Visual Science (supplement) 29,* 43.

Loshin, D. S., & Juday, R. D. (in press). The programmable remapper: Clinical applications for individuals with field defects. *Optometry and Vision Science.*

Schuchard, R. A., & Rubin, G. S. (1989). Face identification of banpass filtered faces by low vision observers. *Investigative Ophthalmology and Visual Science (supplement) 30,* 396.

Chapter 3

FUTURES FOR FAMILIES OF VISUALLY IMPAIRED CHILDREN

Judith Stotland

I am particularly glad that the title of my talk refers to families in the plural, since my first concern is that we all recall that this is anything but a homogenous group. We are rich, we are poor, we are well or poorly educated; we live in cities and on farms; we are of every imaginable religious and cultural background. In fact, one of the best surprises I have had since becoming David's mother is the special friendships I have made with parents with whom I never would have spoken had we not experienced this unique bond. While I am predicting some changes in the sociological mix, it is vital to recall at the outset that each family member of a visually impaired child is every bit as unique in strengths and weaknesses, abilities and needs, as are the students themselves.

I believe that the families of visually impaired children in the year 2014 will be younger, poorer, and far more likely to be from what are now minority cultures in this country. I believe that the children themselves are more likely to be multihandicapped. I further believe that the skills and support that parents need will be the same, but that the modes of delivery will have to be far different.

There are many assumptions underlying these predictions. With a Bush administration in power as our most liberal Supreme Court justices exceed 80 years of age, it is reasonable to assume that court decisions will have an increasingly conservative bent. Nonetheless, I am assuming that abortion will remain legal, although probably not so available at public expense. I further assume that medical technology and treatment will progress in the areas of identifying genetic causes, and possible prenatal correction of certain causes of blindness. Already it is not unusual for an infant with cataracts to have surgery and contact lenses, and for you never to have him or her identified as a potential client! The incidence and impact of congenital glaucoma, which along with cataracts were the twin causes of impairment in my own son, have also been significantly reduced in the past 15 years, and we can expect similar progress in other areas even if we cannot at this time specify which causes of impairment will be reduced. Medical advances have also, however, expanded a different population: low-birthweight babies have produced a growing ROP [retinopathy of prematurity] population, and I do not believe that this problem will be resolved by 2014. If anything, I think it will increase as abortion becomes less available to the poorer segments of society, who are further afflicted with less opportunity for adequate nutrition and prenatal care, although we can hope that the Kennedy initiative for prenatal and early childhood care and nutrition will pass and be adequately funded. I further think that professionals will be seeing a fairly large population of drug babies, although I pray that we will be seeing that group as graduating from the educational system and not a renewing problem in the next 25 years. We know that children with these diagnoses are usually multihandicapped. Currently, preschool workers are reporting 60 percent of their students as multihandicapped; I shouldn't be surprised to see that figure increase significantly. We must be vigilant to assure that these children are not abandoned to a totally generic service delivery, and you must hone your skills to find creative means to meet their needs.

On a more optimistic note, families in the year 2014 who are trying to decide what to do if they are told that they will be having a handicapped child should be receiving a far more positive view of what that child's life can be. A shrinking work force coupled with dramatic demonstrations in the areas of supported employment and mainstreaming should yield families who probably know successfully functioning handicapped adults and former classmates, although they still might never have met a visually impaired person. Each neonatal ICU [intensive care unit] should have a video library with tapes made by parents and handicapped adults speaking about how they cope and the positive quality of their lives. A telephone network should also be in place so that parents could talk directly to others who have children with a similar diagnosis, and with education and rehabilitation specialists who can ensure that parental decisions will be well informed.

Futurists are predicting that by the year 2000, California will be a state where the minorities will be in the majority. Children of immigrants from Third World countries where ophthalmology is either a luxury or nonexistent will be represented beyond their numbers in the visually impaired population. I had assumed that a growing need to be sensitive to multicultural issues will be necessity for specialists in the field who intended to serve in urban areas, but not necessarily in rural states. A recent trip to Iowa reminded me that children are being adopted from other countries, that people settle everywhere, and that multicultural training is indeed a national issue.

Families are likely to be poorer and even more likely than present not to contain a parent not working outside the home, first because we are all predicted to have a lowered lifestyle. Secondly, even the 20 percent share of cost of most current medical insurance can break the most solidly middle-class family who has a medically involved child. Thirdly, medical ethicists are beginning to wrestle with the fact that there is a finite amount of medical care available and that some of it may be more expensive than society can afford. Some respected thinkers are suggesting we develop a hierarchy of services that can be included in insurance coverage. While I hope that this kind of thinking will not prevail, it must be watched closely. What is happening now, has happened in other countries, and would not be solved by the Kennedy initiative, is reduced freedom to choose a specific doctor or even a specific school of thought regarding what is appropriate medical care for a particular condition. Some parents may opt to expend savings to access medical care outside an HMO [health maintenance organization].

Finally, I assume that families that will see handicaps as more "normal," who are working all day, and have strong family values in their culture will expect their children to live at home and attend neighborhood schools. This will compound the problems for a low-incidence population suffering a severe teacher shortage which will have to work with children of more intense needs.

What the families of 2014 will assuredly have in common with those of 1989 are the need for peer support, the need for information in a form comprehensible to the parent at the point when it is given, the availability of caring professionals, and respect for parental expertise.

The concept of a case coordinator as being defined by the P.L. 99-457 planning process gives us the opportunity to refocus attention on the family's centrality in the education process. In listening to people involved in the planning process, I have been interested to notice that there is a small groundswell to create a new profession of case coordinator or, barring that, to devolve it on either the special education teacher or a social worker. While case coordinators will require special training, we don't have enough personnel for that work, and it is detrimental to the child to locate that pivotal role outside the family in most instances. Our best efforts will be directed toward building those skills in the parents who are the most motivated and longest involved persons, and ultimately to teach those skills to the visually impaired person so that in so far as she is capable, she can become her own case coordinator.

What other tools do we now have that will begin to help us cope with the challenges of 2014? I suggest that the most hopeful are technology, the concept of a transdisciplinary team, flexible scheduling, and exploiting the family as a resource.

Technology will be a vital adjunct to teaching skills in future as now. Greater development and use of devices that can directly translate braille to print and vice versa and can enlarge type do help free teacher time for other uses. Other technology that will help us meet the needs of 2014 is available today. We can't train teachers of the visually impaired and expect them to settle in every rural and suburban area that a visually impaired child is likely to be living. We need ways to create teachers of the visually impaired where the child is located. And what of teacher X, who is great at functional low vision assessments for high schoolers but who is assigned a totally blind preschooler? Well, who says you have to sit in room 413 to learn Implications of Blindness? What if you sat in your local TV stations and learned by interactive satellite classes? What if you made a videotape of a lesson with your student and could get it critiqued by a master teacher in another city?

A vital part of planning for P.L. 99-457 is the concept of a transdisciplinary team for delivery of early childhood services. In this model, experts in early childhood education, special education, speech and language, occupational therapy, etc. share their information and perspectives about the individual child and his service needs, and teach one another how to deliver and/or reinforce skills. This model is promising for all ages of our population, but only if the role of the teacher of the visually impaired is not diluted or lost in the process. It can be a means for delivering more services to students with the fewer staff we are likely to have. It also can mean that VH [visually handicapped] teachers needn't become experts in all the additional handicapping conditions their students might possess.

Flexible scheduling of services can deal with several problem areas. Teachers of the visually impaired should not usually be tutors, but you often are. What if you weren't always there for math time? You might be able to work with the child when her parents are home and be able to instruct them as well, and teach him to make his bed or cook a meal using his real home for real work, which seems to reduce the amount of teaching needed. Using the state school in summer for intense work in daily living skills, study skills, braille, etc. can be both a more palatable experience for parents, and another training ground for geographically isolated teachers who are becoming certified as they work with the child.

If we consider the family as a tool, we need to examine its useful components. Too often we speak about the child and perhaps his mother, and oh yes there probably is a father in there somewhere. Someone said recently that everyone else has brothers and sisters; handicapped kids have siblings. Again, P.L. 99-457 planning can help refocus us in this regard by creating the IFSP [Individualized Family Service Plan], which begins by detailing family strengths and weaknesses. Brothers and sisters are great at spending time coloring using a CCTV [closed-circuit television] instead of having an academic exercise of learning how to write. They are great at reducing socially unacceptable behavior: one "Ugh! That's disgusting!" is worth a dozen formal lessons. The best teacher cannot do as much to enhance a child's progress, and the worst teacher cannot sabotage that effort with the skill and certainty of a parent or sibling. Grandparents and other family and community ties are also potential "assistant teachers."

Finally, parents are an untapped resource for recruiting future teachers. Think about giving credit for life experiences, and in-services that would allow movement upwards from a paraprofessional base, and you give parents a forum to share all that was learned to benefit one child with many others.

Chapter 4

FUTURES IN EDUCATION OF VISUALLY IMPAIRED CHILDREN

Michael J. Bina, Ed. D.

Superintendent, Indiana School for the Blind

While we are preoccupied about the future, it's rather ironic: we really haven't explained the past or resolved our current problems or present realities.

The only thing we can say about the future with any degree of certainty is that it will arrive at a constant rate. That is, 60 seconds per minute; 60 minutes per hour. Until the future does arrive, we need to evaluate what we are currently doing, or not doing, and deal with our present problems. We all can design the future and make it what we want it to be, if we invent now. The future will be shaped by your commissions or omissions, by your interest or apathy. Helen Keller wrote that "science may have found cures for most evils, but it has no remedy for the worst of them all—the apathy of human beings" (Koestler, 1976). Nothing will prevent positive advances in the future more than our disinterest, or complacency.

When we think about the future, we all long for the proverbial crystal ball. We rely on wishful thinking and impractical dreaming, hoping that from the crystal ball we will be able to generate easy answers to our complex problems.

In the movie *Vacation,* the Griswalds never planned but projected too far in the future on how great Wallyworld would be once they got there. The movie was good comedy, but in real life this can be tragedy. We often get a lofty goal in our field and start traveling before we plan our trip. As a result, our destination often doesn't live up to our expectations and we become frustrated and waste a lot of money and student learning time.

We perhaps should take a lesson from Noah. He proactively planned and built a simple ark, as opposed to designing a fancy, complex, technological marvel—and most importantly, he did it when it wasn't raining. His timing was right, he was practical, he used common sense, and he built what the situation demanded—nothing more, nothing less. Noah wasn't worried about things other than the immediate weather forecast and his concern for his non-swimmer friends.

While we would like, or anticipate that things in the future will be different, the chances are that many realities will be very much the same. Technically, our cars today are new and improved Model Ts and haven't changed that much since Henry Ford made his first horseless carriage. We have increased the speed of things, but not necessarily improved the quality of life. In the future, we will have to still put in gas, get tune-ups, buy insurance, and if you drive too fast, and get caught, you'll get speeding tickets.

Thirty years ago, the futurists predicted we'd be living in bubble homes and well-protected environments. Actually, houses haven't changed that much in the past 500 years and we shouldn't expect them to change that much in the future. We'll still have heating and cooling bills, mortgage payments, and we will still be doing our favorite pastime—housecleaning—even though we may have a robot helper.

Our students in 2014 will likely have the same stresses, headaches, obstacles, and opportunities as their counterparts have today—and had 25, 50, even 75 years ago. They all share the same needs to read, write, and compute; to travel and live independently; and to socialize and to develop career skills. However, we continue secretly, unrealistically, and over-optimistically to wish for utopia. There's a saying: "It'll be a nice world if they ever get it finished." Realistically, utopia will never be finished. We will always have torn-up roads, potholes, smog, and traffic jams.

Likewise, service delivery models will not change appreciably. As automobiles and houses of the past and present serve to meet our travel and shelter needs, so too will our service delivery models work in the future—hopefully with necessary forthcoming improvements.

Other realities: Governments will never give generously enough to human service programs when there are militaries to build, space to explore, high-incidence lobbies, special interests, and taxpayer resistance,

Also, because of changes in our values, economics, and the family unit, additional obstacles will confront us as professionals. We sometimes think that we are fighting an uphill battle. In the future, the grade will get even steeper. Statistics show that 50 percent of the children today are born to teenage mothers who give birth to at-risk, critically low-weight children. Single-parent families and high poverty rates in such families, child abuse, suicide, home runaways, and drug and alcohol abuse are expected to increase drastically. Minority teachers and racial and cultural positive role models continue to decline. Over 20 percent white, 40 percent Hispanic, and 50 percent black youngsters live in poverty while government and appropriations decline.

Given these realities, "What can we do?" I propose that six words beginning with C's guide your planning. I picked the letter C because I got mostly C's in school—certainly no A's—very few, very few B's.

The six C's are Caring, Conceptualization, Commitment, Collaboration, Confrontation, and Continuation.

CARING

We all care. But caring about our clients with our hearts is clearly not enough. We need to use our analytical skills. Caring is a passive, albeit positive, emotion, but it will not move the mountains we need. We need to be more active, more assertive, work harder, and work smarter. We need to do something about our field's collective ineptness in the legislative process. We need to get political and learn how to play the game.

Also, we dig trenches rather than build bridges and climb mountains. Rather, we circle our wagons, literally fighting among ourselves, rather than fighting the common enemy—the attitudes of the medical community, employers, the general public, and school staff who haven't accepted our students to the degree to which they are entitled. We are confusing our allies with the real enemy and therefore can't hope to grow and progress. We spend too much time getting even—not enough time on getting ahead.

We need to harmonize our beliefs with NFB [National Federation of the Blind] and among ourselves without the expectation of homogenization or compromising our principles. As it is, without the same song, we have discordant disharmony. It's okay that NFB, AER, [Association for Education and Rehabilitation of the Blind and Visually Impaired], or NAPVI [National Association for Parents of the Visually Impaired] sings soprano, bass, or baritone, respectively—but we must settle on a single caring song, blend our harmonies, get an audience, and sing a song like we have never sung before.

CONCEPTUALIZATION

We cannot effect change if we don't plan for it. Change is a process—not an event. For example, the ignorance of the general public will continue to impact negatively on our funding, acceptance, and opportunities for our students unless we intervene nationally. Sure, we talk about educating these various groups—we talk about it a lot, but after all is said and done, much more is said than done!!

To conceptualize we need to use divergent thinking. We tend to restrict our thinking to what is, to tradition, with great care not to rock the boat. Dr. Corn and I have discussed hiring Lee Iaccoca to evaluate our field using the free enterprise/business model standards. Maybe he could tell us where to scratch—I sometimes think we are scratching where it isn't itching, since our itches just don't seem to go away.

Erroneously, we conceptualize with the mind-set that high technology will solve all our problems. After all the fuss with the Laser Cane, our clients left the high-tech bells and whistles for a tool which more closely resembled a stick than an electronic marvel—that is, the long cane. We have overemphasized high tech at the expense of developing our professionals' high-touch interpersonal skills and our students' social skills. We are teaching content and technology with not enough emphasis being placed on teaching people. We need to emphasize interpersonal first, task second.

COMMITMENT

When I think of commitment, I think of the late Claude Pepper. Up to his very last breath, he was committed to improving the lives of others. He didn't retreat, retire—much less tire—due to old age or poor health. He sacrificed the comforts and luxuries of retirement for his cause, the elderly. Sure we all care, but is anyone in this room more caringly committed than Claude Pepper? It has been said that the difference between a "good" and an "excellent" teacher or administrator or representative is that the "excellent" one, to a significantly great degree, gives a damn to really shape the future! We all need, to a very much greater degree, to give a damn! We have grown too complacent—complacent with mediocrity—complacent with whatever the gravy train leaves us. We must start saying, "I will do something!" rather than "Something must be done!"

Rather than having rational commitments, we have accepted fuzzy, yet catchy buzzwords, flashy bandwagons, and invalidated concepts which promise the quick fix, the easy cookbook, and the surefire method or material that was flung at us as the pendulum swung widely away from perfectly good ideas. We need to realize that bandwagons also go to funerals.

Adopting corporate slogans only results in artificial commitments. We have hoped that by projecting we "are committed to excellence" that we will somehow get there. Adopters of such slogans haven't planned or paid the price with hard work on how we can get to excellence, much less taken the time to define what excellence is. A better theme is "we can do better." Slow, steady growth and progress is better than jumping unrealistically to an ill-defined abstract concept.

We need to think more carefully rather than reactively jerking our knees. Our reactive complaining doesn't solve problems any more than fast movement in a rocking chair is responsible for purposeful movement forward. Sam Rayburn (who, I think, was from Arkansas) used to say that any jackass can kick a barn down, but it takes a skilled, committed, hardworking carpenter to build one.

COLLABORATION

We tend to talk to ourselves and we are forever quoting ourselves. This is field echolalia. It has been said that "No man can be really big who does not read widely outside his field." Also, "beaten paths are for beaten men." We cannot stay on beaten paths and stubbornly ignore knowledge in other fields. We have put our eggs all in one basket. We really shouldn't do this because we don't have many eggs and our basket is small. We chase our own tail. We do need to collaborate with other fields more.

CONFRONTATION

Sometimes, too, we are too polite and not assertive enough. We don't want to offend our colleagues in our close-knit circle. Claude Pepper strongly asserted and he wasn't disliked; he was loved. What we publish takes on the aura of unchallenged gospel. We have sacred cows that we worship and dare not challenge. We need more positive agitators like Dr. Barraga to constructively confront many issues. Unless we risk and confront, we will never reach second or third base, or home plate and score, if we continue enjoying the safety of first.

We also protect our students from confronting their own issues. We enable and overprotect on an institutional level. We really don't give our students or their parents true choices and we remove most of all the risks and challenges which bring out the best in individuals.

CONTINUATION

If we start building more bridges and climbing mountains, we will need to retain the gains by continual hard work and proving our need. I suggest focusing on these critical concerns today so that things will be better in 2014:

1. *Literacy skills.* Nationwide, we are not teaching reading, writing, and computing basic skills as well as we could. Some low vision students have been placed on print-only modes of reading, irrespective of reading speed efficiency, when braille, which has been given second-class status, would be more efficient.

2. *Social skill development.* Unfortunately, we're not committing enough time for social skill training, which we know is a most critical variable of whether a person gets, or retains, a job.

3. *SSI [Supplemental Security Income].* We need to make real work more attractive than the easy dollars of SSI, a work dissentive.

4. *Research.* Our field doesn't seem to be focused on the right research questions. Let's ask some new questions!

5. *Accessibility to print.* We have provided better accessibility and accommodations for wheelchair-bound individuals, but nationally, I think it is intolerable that our students don't get textbooks adapted to meet their needs until perhaps late in the school year when their sighted counterparts get their books on the opening day of school. Why can't the federal government give incentives to publishers who generate print and adapted material simultaneously?

6. *Listening to consumers.* Are we making an effort to listen to consumers? Have we given them a forum to speak? Have we asked about how effective our services are? Is it possible, as some have claimed, that we are meeting our needs and possibly not theirs?

7. *Deficit orientation to IEP [Individualized Education Programs] program development.* We tend to define our students' programs based on their deficits rather than their strengths. We ask the students to be "all that they aren't" rather than "all that they can be." Recently, I heard someone facetiously say that if Jesus Christ were to be evaluated with our present system, we would have focused on the negative, ignoring the propounders of the positive.

    Our students have to fail miserably in order to qualify for more intensive services. We have too many kids hanging on by their fingernails who need help, but until they "hit bottom" and are literal academic and social battlefield casualties, they will stay in their present placement.

8. *"The milk of human kindness."* Is it possible that with some of our students, we are not honest enough and we sugarcoat diagnoses and inflate report cards? The milk of human kindness furthers false hope on the road to upcoming bitter disappointment.

9. *Professional deadwood.* We have weak colleagues who should not have been certified, or were competent but "rusted out" in their jobs. Our administrators need to improve their supervisory skills, chop deadwood, and make staff either "grow, glow, or go." The incompetent teacher often hides behind due process rights. These weak staff, in many cases, are granted more process than is due. I know we have a teacher shortage, but it perhaps needs to be selectively greater.

10. *Underserved students.* We have large numbers of underserved students in programs which are touted as comprehensive programs when in fact they are not intensive enough to meet student needs. Two hours of braille instruction per week—or what's worse, per month—is an injustice. In many cases, we have given too little too late and a strong outcry from parents and consumers will strongly increase in intensity in the future.

    "Are our students and clients better off today than they were 10 years ago and will they be better off in the next 25 years if we continue providing services as we do today?" You answer that question.

11. *Emergency certified staff.* Some states give out emergency credentials for 40-80 percent of the VH [visually handicapped] teachers! How would you feel if you were traveling in a Third World nation and got seriously ill and realized that over 50 percent of the medical doctors in the country were on emergency credentials? Today's underserved students are becoming tomorrow's undereducated adults.

Let's look at *service delivery systems*.

1. The *medical community* continues to be detached from our service delivery efforts. Our ophthalmologists for the most part consider irreversible blindness and low vision as their failure. Many admit they lack the skills and knowledge to make referrals. We need a national initiative to educate the medical community.

2. We provide our *transitional services* too late and end up closing the barn door after the horses have left. In our yearly IEP development process we are myopically looking in one-year short-sighted segments and are fragmenting long-range planning. We need to plan what the students will need in the future with an exit orientation in mind and involve rehabilitation earlier.

3. We have *mainstreamed some students before they have been ready.* We continue to push zealously for integration when, for many kids, this becomes a very restricted, counterproductive environment. Some of these students become uninvolved spectators as opposed to active learners and are literally "isolated islands in the mainstream" who are up the creek without paddles, struggling desperately.

    Likewise, we have some students in residential schools who could be integrated more. Nationally, P.L. 94-142 was passed with the cart preceding the horse in that the principals and regular education teachers were not prepared for our students and not enough money was appropriated to do the job right. We have let others (such as TASH [the Association for Persons with Severe Handicaps]) tell us what is best for our students when they have no knowledge of our kids or clients. What is good for one disability group, isn't necessarily what is best for blind children. Not providing an effective rebuttal to TASH's broad, yet articulate generalizations is having adverse effects on our students.

4. We continue to *argue which service delivery option is superior* irrespective of consideration for individual student needs. We need to stop this counterproductive argument and look at how students can move back and forth benefiting from both opportunities.

5. Through our *lack of cooperation between agencies* and among service delivery options we fragment and cause gaps in our services. Need we be a low-incidence cooperation and coordination field?

6. We all know many of our students process information at slower rates than their peers and more time in school is needed to learn skills of independent living, mobility, etc. We persist in piling on and cramming the regular and compensatory skill classes. Why are we *lock-stepping our students to keep up with their peers*? Peer group is important, but if their self-concepts are wounded in our push for them to keep up, what's all the hurry to give them diplomas?

7. While a chicken in every pot was a realistic goal following the Depression, perhaps it is impractical to expect a *VH program in each district* across the country. Decentralization is good, but given our shortage of teachers and our limited resources, perhaps we need to regionally centralize.

8. *Least-restrictive environment.* Why are we defining the guiding light for educational opportunity in negative semantics. Least?—why not "most?" Restrictive?—why not "productive?" Environment?—why not "setting?" Doesn't "most productive setting" sound most positive and a place where we should educate our children than "least restrictive environment?" LRE [least restrictive environment] is a term semantically worthy of the EPA [Environmental Protection Agency]—but definitely inappropriate for our mission. Most productive setting!

9. We *lack a system of national program evaluation, accreditation, and accountability.* NAC [National Accreditation Council for Agencies Serving the Blind and Visually Handicapped] has not been widely embraced and is still a voluntary service—probably the agencies that need the most careful scrutiny are the ones not asking for accreditation. Why, if teachers have to pass competency tests, aren't agencies and schools required to undergo mandatory accountability scrutiny?

Let's look at *teaching training.*

1. It bothers me that our youth are not interested in being educators. I asked my nephew last summer what he was going to major in in college. His response was business, law, or pre-

med. I asked, "What about education?" By the time he stopped laughing, I realized that we have a real problem in our field. Hopefully, many of the upwardly mobile yuppies will realize the emptiness of the BMW existence and will trade in those BMW's and become the driving forces behind IEP's.

A problem contributing to the teacher shortage may be poor pay. Significant amount of learning time is wasted using substitute teachers. There is no substitute for the teacher. We pay our hourly employees at McDonald's more than our substitute teachers. This makes for fast food, but unfortunately slow learning.

Our teachers have assumed too many new hats of low vision, technology, and multihandicapped specialist, counselor, diagnostician, consultant, inservice trainer, advocate, parent trainer, etc. We have created "generalistic specialists" jacks of all trades, but true masters of none. One person can't have all the competencies, much less cram that much knowledge and skills in the amount of time allowed in traditional training programs. A superintendent colleague was encouraging me to hire a practicum student interning at his school. I asked in what areas can she teach. The response was "everything." Everything?!? I submit if you can teach "everything," you can teach nothing very well!

Dr. Barraga and Dr. Swallow point out that "low vision" was listed #1 as the competency most needed out in the field by two different studies. Yet the curricula in the training programs haven't changed appreciably. Dr. Swallow has some interesting ideas about what we might do in the future. Her national training center proposal and other worthy ideas will be published in an upcoming issue of *RE:view*.

Let's look at our *involvement with parents*.

1. In regular education, President Bush is talking parent choice for school placement. Yet in our yearly conferences, we seldom give parents a true choice. Regular education parents, if they are dissatisfied with an educational program, can opt for private school. The options for our parents are limited. In Indiana, we have a parent option where parents, if they are not pleased with LEA [local education agency] services, can opt for the residential school placement, and vice versa. The parents and students buy in the program with feelings of empowerment and ownership. Parents' choice will be a future reality, and a controversial one.

2. A parent recently told me that the law discriminates, since it specifies "integration with nonhandicapped children." He asked, "Are handicapped peers less valuable than children without handicaps?" Good question! He also asked, "Don't kids with handicaps benefit from interaction with other kids with similar challenges? How dare the social makers tell me who my son's friends will be—or who he can't interact with!" This was good food for thought for me.

3. We need to be more concerned about parent self-image. I hear the phrase all too often that some of our parents don't care. This harsh, quick judgment invalidly and unkindly blames

the parents, the student, and other scapegoats for student failure and lack of progress. We need to scrutinize our own contributions to student failures.

4. Let's talk about you. We will need more social worker skills in dealing with an ever-increasing number of dysfunctional families. While we are seeing more students with head injuries, multi-involvements, and premies due to maternal drugs, poor prenatal care, disease, etc., I don't believe we have seen staff development and preservice programs adjust to the changing caseloads.

In the next 25 years, we will all need to further develop ourselves. Ten years ago, we heard a lot about burnout. We realize that this was more a buzzword than a real phenonomen. There were more symptoms of "rust out," boredom, and lack of challenge. Basically, by not growing and developing and by not getting positively reinforced, morale and effectiveness were lowered.

We all need to invest in ourselves. We need to go back to school. We need to hungrily read from other fields and we need to prime our own pumps and fill our emotional gas tanks. We started out as eager idealists in the field, but with the realities on the job, we became somewhat disillusioned. We need to continue to guard against getting in a rut, becoming discouraged and pessimistic. Remember that in the future if we "lose sight of ourselves while being concerned with our mission, we will be lost, we will lose ourselves and our missions" [author unknown].

I hope that I have provided something of substance which will stimulate your planning this afternoon. I hope that for some, I have inspired you—and the rest of you at least will wake up refreshed!

Congratulations on your 25th!

REFERENCES

Koestler, F. A. (1976). *The unseen minority: A social history of blindness in the United States.* New York: David McKay.

National Center for Health Statistics. (1990). *Obesity in children.* Washington, DC: Author.

Chapter 5

FUTURES IN ASSESSMENT: THE LEARNING ENVIRONMENT FOR STUDENTS WITH LOW VISION

Susan Jay Spungin, Ed. D.

Associate Executive Director
Program Services
American Foundation for the Blind

When Dr. Corn first approached me to speak at this Symposium, I was both flattered and pleased to be asked to share in the celebration of the twenty-fifth anniversary of the low vision program at the University of Texas at Austin. What a compliment to be included and what an opportunity to spend time considering the future—some twenty-five years from now—the year 2014. Twenty-five is also a symbolic number for me personally and professionally, for it was twenty-five years ago at age 23 that I started my career as a musician-turned-teacher of the visually handicapped thanks to my friend and mentor Georgie Lee Abel. And, God willing, with medical science at my back I will still be involved in the year 2014 at age 73! Admittedly perhaps from home with grandchildren and great-grandchildren competing for my time.

As I began to organize my thoughts and resources for this presentation, I saw clearly that this was no easy assignment. Should I approach the year 2014 as what the ideal should be or with what a heavy sense of cynical Northeastern upbringing tells me it realistically might be? As my friend and colleague, Mary Ellen Mulholland, AFB [American Foundation for the Blind]'s Director of AFB Press would say, before we can predict the future, we must know where we are in the present, and by understanding the present we can determine the future need and plan for it accordingly. A wise thought but a difficult task indeed.

Well, where are we in the present? From my perspective, we are a nation that still gives lip service to the needs of the minority and disabled population and a federal government that continues to respond more to the power of numbers than to specific separate, yes, categorical special needs of the low-incidence group of disabled individuals, in our case the totally blind and low vision person.

In the field of education for the blind and low vision student, we continue to be unable to determine how to define uniformly our population both in terms of functional versus clinical acuity measures as well as appropriate service delivery models. We continue to be so worried over issues of turf that the consumer movement has developed almost around us, touching us only minimally. I believe many of us are distrustful of the consumer movement and spend more time listening for supposed hidden agenda than to its actual message. A message, ironically, we agree with more times than not. We are a profession that since the 60s has had to fight for the first time for resources for the visually handicapped population, competing with other groups of disabled people and trying to save many of our legislative victories won during the first half of the twentieth century. I believe many have never become used to this competition for resources at the federal and state level and have dealt with it from a state of passivity to "it won't happen in my backyard" attitude. Even today, I see programs and actions that continue to rearrange the deck chairs on the Titanic, giving little thought to new innovative ways of thinking and planning—not for the future but for now. Because if we don't truly start to problem solve the many issues facing us today, I fear for our future. With no trained teachers of the visually handicapped or O&M [orientation and mobility] instructors available to hire, what is the Director of Special Education to do? With no data to document numbers and need, how is the legislator, state or federal, to help? And finally, the scandal of the blindness field's disunity among its consumers and providers continues to retard our growth.

Where are the professional risk takers and daredevils of the decades of the 40s, 50s and early 60s? We have historically been the first and the leaders in so many areas. The first to integrate or mainstream students who were visually impaired, the first to truly translate research into practice—low vision being one of several examples of this. The first to consider technology as a viable part of a child's curriculum and teacher training programs from Optacons to Speech Plus calculators. The first to accept the responsibility for multihandicapped blind children such as deaf-blind and other populations. The first to have university preparation programs develop in relative consensus and implement a competency-based teacher training model for teacher-educators to tailor to their own curriculum structures. Perhaps it was "the best of times" that allowed for our enormous growth but looking back, I'm not sure if it was always the best of times. The Vietnam War, campus unrest, political assassinations, flower power, women's liberation, the black movement, and the beginning of a Watergate mentality. I'm not sure I would characterize that always the best of times—although we did put a man on the moon.

What will be the social context of the year 2014? What will the general population look like? By the year 2080, it is projected that Hispanics will comprise 19.2 percent of the population, blacks 17.9 percent, with the Asian-American population the third largest ethnic minority. The number of married couples with children will continue to decline and presently represents only 25 percent of all households. By the year 1995, married couples without children is projected at 52.5 percent, and families and households headed by men at 7.5 percent. In fact, today only 7 percent of families are made up of married couples with children where the husband is the sole provider. The impact the changing family structure will have on child care and early intervention programs seems obvious.

America's teaching force is undergoing many changes as well. Many of the older, more experienced teachers are retiring (some 36 percent by 1995) and many newer younger teachers are leaving for other occupations. Fewer college graduates are choosing teaching as a career. These changes, combined with the expected rise of the number of school-age children from the new-collar class of baby boomlets, low pay and prestige, and high stress, all point to severe shortages now and in the future. A shortage of college professors is also predicted, with almost 40 percent of the nation's college faculty retiring by the year 2000. In addition, the Carnegie Foundation suggests that low salaries may prompt 40 percent more of college professors to leave their profession.

The corporation as a teacher, a new phenomenon, started in the 1980s, is truly a reflection of the corporate perception that the traditional education system in America is failing, leaving corporations with the task of educating their work force. In 1990 it is projected that the number of students enrolled will be equal to those attending four-year college or university training programs. If this proves true, teachers and vocational educators for the visually impaired population have to become much more closely aligned with industry and the corporate sector.

The last trend I will highlight due to time constraints is generational equality, an issue that has a potential for conflict based on the growing numbers of the elderly. According to the principles of generational equality, society should not advocate for one age or generation without considering the competing rights and claims of others. Looking at it simplistically, I believe the aging low vision person may have the political power to improve health care and eye care in general due to the large numbers alone, and it may help young children as well, both in terms of financial support and access to new treatments and practices.

Let's now look at some data on estimated prevalence of persons with low vision. A 57 percent growth rate of low vision elderly from 1986 to the year 2015 above the age of 65 is predicted. One must also note the 45-64 age group increasing by 73 percent as a result of the baby boom. This certainly indicates increased issues pointing toward the need in employment readiness skills as well as in the development of creative employment opportunities. In general terms, we will see a 17 percent increase over the age group of under 18, but I caution you as to the underreporting of this group in particular—a function of the questionable survey techniques of the 1977 Health Interview on which these are based. However, in general terms, looking at the overall demographic composition, the year 2014 holds for us a great increase in numbers of low vision people, especially above the age of 65. If the totally blind were included in this data, it is estimated that the percent change would be 2 percent higher in each of the age groups.

The remainder of the presentation will attempt to focus specifically on assessing the learning environment of low vision people in the year 2014 and the impact that it will have on teachers of the visually handicapped. Let me preface these remarks by saying I have tried to be controversial in order to take literally the task assigned—that being to stimulate your thinking in a way that allows you to project the probable skills and resource needs of the visually handicapped person in the year 2014. I have attempted to scan the environments of legislative development, medical advances and school and home community along with skills needed by teachers of the visually handicapped. What I have left out is the low vision person but have the following to offer in this area by way of background.

I predict by the year 2014, our nation will have reorganized the school year to approximate the Japanese structure of longer days and an 11-month program year. It may be required to add a 13th year to allow extra time for some students to pass a rigorous competence-based final exam taken senior year requiring expert knowledge in math and science as well as communication skills. There will be a national required school accreditation program—generally based in general education but with categorical standards applied by professionals in low incidence programs, i.e., visually handicapped, deaf and hard of hearing, physically handicapped and English as a second language programs.

The extended school day and year will be fought by the unions, possibly requiring an increase in teachers and/or greater compensation. The mandated age of 16 to attend school will be moved to 18 for regular education. Advanced technical vocational schools, corporate training, and colleges and universities will be more heavily attended, since blue-collar jobs requiring minimal skills will be few in number.

This has been both a fun and difficult presentation to prepare because many of my predictions I do not wish for, where many others I do. By the year 2014, we will have seen two new presidents, assuming each tenure is eight years. Perhaps by the year 2008 minority group leadership in politics will be commonplace. What will that do to my predictions? Which of my predictions are most likely and which really could make a difference? How many "wild cards" such as the AIDS epidemic will happen between now and 2014? Time will tell. But the reality remains that if we want change for or against a trend we must take steps far in advance to support or oppose changes in our environment to assure our voices are heard. We need to have more symposiums like this one in order to more closely focus on future needs against future realities so we can become prepared and effective advocates for ourselves and services, not to mention the low vision individuals we care about.

Thank you.

I. LEGISLATIVE ENVIRONMENT

ENVIRONMENT

1. P.L. 99-457 - earlier I.D. [identification of visually impaired children].

2. P.L. 94-142 — 37 years old.

3. IEP [Individualized Education Program] for all children.

4. TB [Talking Books] program taken over by for profit.

5. APH [American Printing House for the Blind] includes technology from outside under quota — drops L.P. [large-print] books — reallocates money.

6. NIB [National Industries for the Blind] goes generic due to MH/VH [multiply handicapped/visually handicapped] and growth of supportive employment and work enclaves.

7. Parent groups and individual rights stronger.

8. P.L. 89-313 funds under P.L. 94-142 and residential schools tied more closely to public school programs.

9. Title VIC reclassifies D/B [deaf-blind] as MH [multiply handicapped].

TEACHER OF VISUALLY HANDICAPPED

1.2.3. Integrating LV [low vision] instruction into entire curriculum for all LV children including recreational activities, etc. Child care and early intervention programs for visually impaired children are required to have specially certified teachers.

4. Heavy emphasis on listening skills in all grades.

5. Good contrast magnification for maps and graphs by adapting materials easily with good photocopy equipment.

6. Job site evaluation and work modifications with vocational education will increase. Computers are equalizers but negative attitudes of employers and others remain a problem.

7. Flexible work hours allowing for teacher conferences with parents after school or on weekends since both are working parents.

8. Teach independence education to include social skills, problem solving, and advocacy.

9. Sophisticated assessments allow the effects of vision to be distinguished from other disabilities present in the multiply handicapped child.

(continued)

I. LEGISLATIVE ENVIRONMENT (*continued*)

10. Better demographic data due to computer technology and data base networking.

11. A system of national program evaluation, accreditation, and accountability through NAC [National Accreditation Council for Agencies Serving the Blind and Visually Handicapped] is implemented fully nationwide.

10. Easier tracking of children and child find allowing for better program planning in advance. Computer data base access to all titles and materials needed for VH children combines lists of APH, LC [Library of Congress], RFB [Recording for the Blind], and IMCVH [Instructional Materials Centers for the Visually Handicapped] centers.

11. Teachers of VH will have some measure of accountability and source for best practice.

II. MEDICAL ENVIRONMENT

ENVIRONMENT

1. Prevention of some diseases, especially those inherited, i.e., RP [retinitis pigmentosa], etc.—gene splicing.

2. Retinal transplants.

3. Surgery improves low vision and blindness.

4. Contact lens technology allows for greater corrective bifocal contacts with greater magnification.

5. Diagnostic techniques allow for earlier intervention of eye disorders.

6. Low vision devices attractive and cost covered under health plan(s)—third party payment for LV [low vision] service and devices.

7. Ophthalmologists recognize LV as a specialty and develop with others a scope and sequence of courses. Also, then refer to LV specialists.

TEACHER OF VISUALLY HANDICAPPED

1.2.3. Computers developed and able to interpret brain waves in order for professionals to simulate visual experiences of their students/clients in terms of how the consumer sees the environment, making functional assessment a thing of the past. An increased understanding of brain and neurological functioning as it relates to sight and seeing has resulted in improved methods of teaching the VI [visually impaired].

4. Greater understanding of optics.

5. Better assessment tools on LV and greater validity and reliability allow greater precision - functional assessments.

6. Greater understanding of psychosocial aspects of devices and sensory input.

7.8. Due to technological advances for congenitally and adventitiously involved persons, greater numbers of VI people have been medically improved. As a result, vision rehabilitation and LV specialists have emerged as a separate profession from special education.

(continued)

II. MEDICAL ENVIRONMENT (*continued*)

8. Due to advances, congenital and adventitious blind see and LV can be medically improved—vision rehabilitation becomes a necessary service. LV and vision rehabilitation specialist services are covered by insurance and health care providers as a part of standard medical practice because the increased political power of the aging VI population has resulted in enhanced financial support for health and eye care for VI children. Increased prevalence of LV among the aging population has resulted in greater acceptance of individuals with VI [visual impairments]. Socialized health systems exist and result in prompt referral and appropriate services as standard practice for VI.

III. SCHOOL AND HOME ENVIRONMENT

ENVIRONMENT

1. Electronic blackboards—individual instruction.

2. Speech technology everywhere (OCR [optical character recognition]—talking yellow pages, captioning movies, video texts for plays, portable personal reader, money identifier, etc. - speech technology, multilingual and more human sounding.

3. "Smart homes"—voice recognition for controlling environment, communication, and security.

4. More adaptable lighting for professional and personal use.

5. Display technology progresses to point of being flat, high contrast, needing little power, and portable. With cameras to be inexpensive, portable (CCTVs [closed-circuit televisions]).

6. Environmental simulators, like those used in flight training, have standardized O&M [orientation and mobility] instruction for those with LV [low vision].

7. Automatic bank teller machines and other graphic displays have been converted to large print and/or speech output for greater access to the VI [visually impaired].

TEACHER OF VISUALLY HANDICAPPED

1. More a consultant than teacher in most cases.

2. Listening skills emphasized and teachers are bilingual.

3.4.5. Develop for students greater flexibility to work and move among various media systems.

6. Develop with O&M a set curriculum to teach O&M to LV students.

7.8.9. Knowledgeable in the teaching of a variety of technological devices and selected software systems for self-instructional programs for in-service individuals as well as for LV students.

10. Case manager model with multidisciplinary approach - LV core of competencies for VI and MH [multiply handicapped] and other areas of special education.

11. Teaching becomes a competitively attractive profession.

12. Categorical teacher preparation funding available, with generous living stipends in order to recruit teachers.

13. Greater diagnostic and remedial teaching skills.

(continued)

III. SCHOOL AND HOME ENVIRONMENT (*continued*)

8. Physical location of all public-use machines or buildings barrier free.

9. Greater use of military technology: night vision, electronic imaging sensors.

10. Itinerant and consulting model continues most popular with resource and special classes more generic and for MH/VH [multiply handicapped/visually handicapped]. Disability labels a thing of the past, requiring a greater need for assessment skills to be functionally based, tailored to categorical needs of blind and LV students.

11. Esteem of teaching profession raised, along with salaries.

12. Special education credentials require 30 units beyond a master's in general secondary or elementary education.

13. Master's in general education required for all teachers, with infused teaching methods for learning disabled, so this group is no longer seen as a separate category of disabled.

Table 1

ESTIMATED PREVALENCE OF PERSONS WITH LOW VISION IN
THE U.S., 1986 AND 2015*

Age (in years)	Estimated Prevalence of Persons with Low Vision**		% Change
	YEAR		
	1986	2015	
ALL AGES	2,762,100	4,279,000	+55
Under 18	31,300	36,500	+17
18-44	123,900	109,600	-12
45-64	261,100	451,400	+73
65-74	810,900	1,171,300	+44
75+	1,534,900	2,510,200	+64
* *
65+	2,345,800	3,681,500	+57

Prepared by: Katherine A. Nelson, Social Research Department, American Foundation for the Blind, June 6, 1989.

*"Low vision" is defined here as severe visual impairment (the inability to read ordinary newspaper print even with correction) that does *not* involve total blindness.

**For age groups under 65, the estimates for both years use [the National Center for Health Statistics's] 1977 National Health Interview Survey rates, the latest year for which information on severe visual impairment was obtained for the whole sample. For the age groups 65 and older, the rates were obtained from Supplement on Aging to the 1984 Healthy Interview Survey, which employed improved interview techniques. For all age groups, the appropriate rates were applied to population estimates by the U.S. Bureau of the Census.

To exclude totally blind people from our estimates, we used rates from 1970 found in *Vision Problems in the U.S.,* published by NSPB [National Society to Prevent Blindness].

BIBLIOGRAPHY

Books And Periodicals

A nation prepared: Teachers for the 21st century. (1986, May). Carnegie Forum on Education and the Economy.

Bishop, V. E. (1988). Making choices in functional vision evaluations: Noodles, needles, and haystacks. *Journal of Visual Impairment & Blindness, 82,* 94-99.

Corn, A. L. (1985). An independence matrix for visually handicapped learners. *Education of the Visually Handicapped, 17* (1), 3-10.

Corn, A. L. (1986). Low vision and visual efficiency. In G. T. Scholl (Ed.), *Foundations of education for blind and visually handicapped children and youth: Theory and practice* (pp. 99-117). New York: American Foundation for the Blind.

Corn, A. L. (1989). Instruction in the use of vision for children and adults with low vision: A proposed program model. *RE:view, 21* (1), 26-39.

Managing how for the 1990's. (1988, September 26). *Fortune.*

On the threshold of independence: A report to the president and congress of the United States. (1988, January). National Council on the Handicapped.

What lies ahead: Looking toward the 90's. (1987). United Way.

Much appreciation is given to the staff at the American Foundation for the Blind (AFB) who helped me brainstorm many ideas found in this paper.

Dr. Kathleen Huebner, Director, National Services in Education, Low Vision, and Orientation and Mobility

Dr. Corinne Kirchner, Director, Social Research

Ms. Katherine Nelson, Senior Research Associate

Ms. Leslye Piqueras, National Consultant in Low Vision

Ms. Leslie Rosen, AFB Librarian

Mr. Elliot Schreier, Director, National Technology Center

Dr. Alana Zambone, National Consultant in Early Childhood and Multi-Disabilities

Chapter 6

REPORTS OF THE SESSION LEADERS

SESSION 1. Leader: Dr. Virginia Bishop

The statement of concern was: "Service delivery systems and teaching methodologies for visually impaired in the year 2014 have not changed appreciably from the standard practices of 1989." Since the group considered this statement to be an undesirable outcome, it viewed the concepts of facilitator and inhibitor in reverse; that is, a facilitator was a factor that would support the *undesired* result, and an inhibitor was a force that would produce a *desired* change. To simplify the discussion, factors were listed as those that would "make it happen" and those that would "keep it from happening." This portion of the futures process produced two lists of factors as follows:

Facilitators	*Inhibitors*
1. No funding.	1. More multiply handicapped children.
2. Rigid school administrators.	2. More technology.
3. Shortages of VH [visually handicapped] teachers.	3. New laws.
4. Lack of ongoing in-services.	4. New research—practical and applied—research into practice.
5. Low incidence/prevalence of the population.	5. Knowledgeable supervision.
6. High caseloads.	6. Outreach resource assistance.
7. General public attitudes.	7. Stronger consumer voice.
8. Geographic area required of itinerant teachers.	8. Greater interagency cooperation.
9. Lack of peer interaction (professionals).	9. Better transitional planning—birth to death.
10. Ineffective regional service delivery.	10. Expanded definition of visually handicapped.

11. Lack of consistency in methodologies (variations between programs, states, etc.), funding, etc.

12. Ineffective child identification and tracking system.

11. More comprehensive teacher education and outreach programs.

12. Financial support and time release for advanced training.

13. Appropriate pay for time and responsibility.

14. Practical/innovative experiences in teacher education.

15. "Real teachers" brought in on panels during training courses.

It was recognized that many of these factors were interrelated and difficult to address as individual issues. However, to facilitate the futures process, the group selected five factors as the most critical—three facilitators and two inhibitors. The group was unable to agree on weights for the factors, so it assigned arbitrary weights of 20 points each. (Theoretically, therefore, the statement of concern would be gradually steered toward occurrence, an undesired outcome.)

To select a point of entry, the group rank-ordered the five factors (from most to least important) as follows:

1. Ineffective child identification and tracking system
2. Shortage of VH teachers
3. No funding
4. More comprehensive teacher education and outreach programs
5. New research, practical and applied.

Strategies for change were suggested for each factor. (The session leader proposed that the concept of unlimited monetary resources should guide the group's thinking, so that creative solutions could be advanced for the apparent problems.) It appeared that an accurate identification and tracking system (for students) was the prime requisite for change. Without this system there is no basis on which to project the need for personnel, programs, or funding. Suggestions for implementing such a system included a consistent referral process (definition, procedure, central repository of data) and a central, national, computerized data bank. The repository for the data could include the National Institutes of Health or the American Foundation for the Blind; the data-collection method could utilize procedures followed by the U.S. Bureau of the Census.

The shortage of teachers of visually impaired students was the second factor to be considered. The primary difficulty seemed to be the lack of interest in teaching as a profession and the lack of definition for a teacher of visually impaired students. Therefore, the group proposed that a public relations–public awareness campaign was needed to build the image of the teacher of visually impaired students and to enhance the desirability of the teaching profession, in general. There seemed to be a consensus that increased salaries for special teachers would provide additional incentive to enter the field.

Lack of funding was the third concern. Since most of the older problems were directly related to the availability (or unavailability) of funds, strategies for influencing this area were of great importance. Two strategies that were suggested were lobbying of legislators (and the public) and exploring private funding sources (e.g., foundations and corporations) for financial support.

The group considered the status of teacher education programs to be a major factor in preventing the undesirable outcome of the original statement. It was felt that distance training (e.g., courses provided via television, telephone, or other forms of technology) was one viable method of taking teacher education *to* prospective teachers of visually impaired students (rather than waiting for them to come to the college or university campus). Another variation on this theme was the endorsement of outreach courses. An additional suggestion was that the sequence of courses to prepare and certify teachers should be expanded and, if necessary, lengthened. The group thought that more specific course work was needed in such areas as early childhood, multiple handicaps, public relations, counseling, and technology to prepare teachers to meet the needs of the changing population of students and the evolving society.

The final area of concern was research. The group proposed a central clearinghouse for information, where individual teachers could telephone or write for assistance on specific problems. This central resource was viewed as a depository of current research and state-of-the-art expertise and a networking clearinghouse (i.e., a hot line for problem solving). An additional concern expressed by the group was that teachers have limited opportunities to receive training in the applications of new research and that this needed to be addressed, since research was deemed to be of limited value unless it could be used to improve methodology or expand expertise.

The unaddressed factors were no less important forces for change, but the brief time allotted for this session only permitted exploration of the five factors discussed above. The remaining forces are left to the reader (or a group of responders with more time) to analyze.

SESSION 2. Leader: Dr. Marcia Moore

The group was given two high likelihood–high impact events as choices for discussion and chose the following statement for examination: "Child care and early intervention programs for visually impaired children are required to have specially certified teachers." The group brainstormed 14 separate ideas that it eventually collapsed into seven. Before it organized these factors, however, it established certain definitions. *Child care* was defined as preschool or nursery school, *not* day care. *Early intervention* was described as home-based–center-based mixed-model services. *Certification* was determined to be certification in visual impairments plus early childhood training (similar to the certification described in the recommendations made by the CEC [Council for Exceptional Children] Certification Committee in 1986-87).

Facilitators listed were:

30 POINTS 1. Legislative impact (including enforcement and monitoring of legislation, and the continuation of P.L. 99-457, especially as it applies to the parental involvement in the Family Service Plan design and delivery).

Inhibitors listed were:

30 POINTS 1. Funding resources to provide salary increase, preservice training, and university-based training programs; insufficient number of available people/professionals.

20 POINTS 2. Certification and training (including the defining of required certification [ECE/ECSE vs. VH (early childhood education/early childhood special education vs. visually handicapped)] and in-service training [ECE, VH, multicultural, MH (multiply handicapped), etc.].

10 POINTS 3. Research regarding the effects of early intervention programs.

5 POINTS 4. Philosophy of agencies relative to service delivery systems (center vs. home-based and parent component).

3 POINTS 5. Location: rural vs. urban.

2 POINTS 6. Attitudes (both public and political).

NOTE: Although both legislation and funding received an equal number of points, the group prioritized legislation before funding.

Strategies for implementing positive change were developed. To create a legislative impact, the group thought that three steps would be needed:

1. Mobilization/education of parents for legislative advocacy through in-service programs, parent support groups, and/or associations (e.g., NAPVI [National Association for Parents of the Visually Impaired]).

2. Monitoring by teachers associations (e.g., AER [Association for Education and Rehabilitation of the Blind and Visually Impaired], CEC [Council for Exceptional Children]) of compliance to enforce existing legislation.

3. Advocacy by parents and professionals.

To deal with the funding problem, several strategies were suggested:

1. Salary increases could be obtained through coalitions of teachers, nurses, and social workers in agencies; grass-roots lobbying of legislators for educators' salaries; contracting with specialists in visual impairment who are in private practice; and lobbying for incentive programs and stipends.

2. To address the lack of trained people, parents could be trained as paraprofessionals and given credit and career-ladder incentives to encourage them to become professionals.

3. Training programs could be funded cooperatively by school districts; preservice training could be given in exchange for a commitment to work a specific number of years.

To address the problems of certification and training, several ideas were advanced:

1. First determine which type of certification is most needed—EC or VH; a compromise may be indicated because of the lack of time or money. Certification in EC or ECSE plus VH would be ideal.

2. Require course work on visual impairments for EC teachers who have visually impaired children in their classes.

3. Require a consultant on visual impairment to be available and involved if a visually impaired child is in a class.

4. Utilize creative technology, such as interactive television and videotapes, to provide in-service training.

5. In-service training should be multicultural, based on the population (or anticipated population) to be served.

SESSION 3. Leader: Dr. Rita Livingston

Two statements were assigned to this group, but only one was explored in any great depth. The first statement was: "Automatic bank teller machines and other graphic displays have been converted to large print and/or speech output for greater access to the visually impaired." The group thought that evidence already existed to suggest that this objective is currently being achieved. Canada has speaking teller machines in some areas of the country; the United States and other countries have speaking electronic scanners in such places as supermarkets. Although the group recognized the need for continued development and implementation on a broader basis for this event, they chose to concentrate their statement exploration on the second event statement: "Reductions in cost and size of low vision aids, along with added versatility, have permitted these aids to be 'programmed' to meet individual needs, pathologies, and/or tasks." A random list was generated of factors related to this concept. At the completion of the "brainstorming" session, each factor was identified as a facilitator or inhibitor, as follows:

Facilitators identified:

1. Government support of development (money and personnel should be available to develop programmable devices). Some work in this area is already being done.

2. Adopt or adapt technology from other disciplines, rather than "reinventing the wheel." We need to look at devices available in other fields/disciplines; some devices may be usable as they exist, and can be adopted; others may need minor or perhaps even major revisions before being applicable. Despite the need for revisions, initial development costs will be saved.

3. Mass production techniques are available; consider production outside the United States for cost reasons. Convert this type of technology into toy markets, or look at toy markets and adapt. This approach could increase productivity and market numbers of lower costs.

4. Industry/business need to be encouraged to provide/promote the use of technology among workers and within facilities.

5. If applicable to cultural/economic structure of countries outside the United States, devices should be promoted there as well.

6. Statewide networking should be developed, put in place, and functioning.

7. Accumulate knowledge of consumer opinions/wishes. There is some information already available, and capabilities exist to gather more information through surveys (mail, telephone, electronic media). Consideration needs to be given to consumer wants/needs; the cosmetics of devices need to be considered to make them least obtrusive/noticeable. Factors for acceptance must be explored for consumers, in particular, and also for other groups (e.g., employers, families, etc.). The effects on self-concept of consumers is critical to the successful use of devices, and may be the *most* critical factor of all. Little, if any, attention has been paid to effects on family members (their concept of the consumer and the effects of those concepts on the consumer).

Inhibitors identified:

1. The lack of monetary support to the consumer of these devices puts them out of reach of the vast majority of individuals (school-age children as well as adults).

2. Lack of sophistication on the part of legislators could inhibit the development of special devices. Efforts need to be made to inform legislators about consumer need, cost efficiency of programmed devices, and lifelong effects upon consumers.

3. Transdisciplinary use of technology will be needed; territorialism currently creates problems.

4. The consumer is often uninformed about new technology or devices.

Strategies seemed to emerge as part of the factors. Some of them were isolated into statements, although weighting was not accomplished. Many of the group thought that *all* factors were of equal weight, and no consensus could be reached on the weighting. The following strategies seemed to be important to the group:

1. Survey existing technology, especially that in other fields, to determine whether any devices can be adopted as is or adapted to meet the needs of visually impaired individuals.

2. Create an incentive for employers to provide and/or promote the use of special devices in the workplace.

3. Survey consumers to determine what *they* want, need, and would use; determine the impact of a variety of devices on the consumer (e.g., self-esteem, cosmetic) and his/her family.

4. Provide funds to consumers, to help them purchase special devices.

5. Educate legislators about consumer needs and the cost-effectiveness of special devices in terms of productivity.

6. Promote the use of devices across disciplines, to minimize the "specialness" of such devices.

7. Devise a program to inform consumers about what is already available. Construct training programs to assist consumers to learn how to use devices and what to do if the devices malfunction. (If the consumer does not know what to do to secure repair of a malfunctioning device, it may have an effect on the long-term acceptance of the device.)

SESSION 4. Leader: Dr. Sandy Parsons

This session's topic statement was "The knowledge of how visually impaired children learn has doubled; therefore, vision teachers devote more service delivery time to teaching the use of available vision." Although there was considerable discussion about the relationship between the first half of the statement and the second (i.e., would increased knowledge of how visually impaired children learn reduce time spent in instructional skills and increase emphasis on increasing visual efficiency, or are the two parts of the statement unrelated, or are they related only in terms of teaching methodology?), it was decided that the discussion should focus on both aspects but not necessarily on implied relationships. The group thought that it would be desirable to know more about how visually impaired children learn and that it would also be desirable to spend more time teaching the use of available vision, but it is important to understand more about how *all* children learn.

Since the issues were somewhat broadly stated, it was difficult to define clear forces. Despite these difficulties, the following forces were identified; weights were assigned to the forces felt by the group to be most critical.

Restrainers:

1. Heterogeneity of the group;
2. Rural America; and
3. Generic trends in education (10 points).

Facilitators

1. Appropriate caseloads for teachers;
2. Increased funding/resources/services (35 points);
3. Role release of professionals; attitude change;
4. Research/technology (25 points); and
5. Improved quality of personnel preparation programs (30 points).

The group determined that the facilitators outweighed the restrainers, with the resulting probability that the event statement would occur unassisted. However, a number of strategies were suggested by the group, to *ensure* the event's occurrence.

Strategy 1: Increase public awareness.

The group felt that several factors should be considered in increasing public awareness. There had to be a dissemination of information about the uniqueness of the visually impaired population. The public also had to be informed about the critical shortage of personnel in the field. A final element in this strategy was the cost-benefit ratio, which meant that taxpayers had to be informed that expenditures would prove their long-term value in terms of employability and productivity of visually impaired persons.

Strategy 2: Cooperation as a field, in fund raising.

The group recognized that there were a great many disconnected fund-raising efforts in the vision field. They also recognized that more cooperative efforts might yield better results.

Strategy 3: More efficient use of funds and resources, through interagency cooperation.

The group agreed that "turf-protection" among agencies generally resulted in inefficient use of funds/resources and duplication of services. A better application of both funds and resources might result from interagency cooperation.

Strategy 4: Incorporation of the family into service delivery.

It was recognized by the group that families may be an underutilized source of support and that their role in service delivery could be expanded. Although parents were intended by law to be an important part of the educational process, they often played a minor role in reality. The responsibilities of the vision teacher could be greatly reduced if parents and families could be enlisted to provide follow-through on instructional goals. Such support could shift teacher time and emphasis to other disability-related areas (e.g., the "teaching of the use of available vision").

Strategy 5: Training and use of volunteers.

Since time spent with students appeared to be a factor in the issues, some discussion by the group suggested that a possible solution might be the use of volunteers. Some training of these volunteers would be essential, but the time spent would be repaid in terms of teacher release time for other more essential teaching responsibilities.

Strategy 6: Increased funding, resources, and services.

The most critical factors that recurred repeatedly in the discussion were funding, resources availability, and service delivery. It was recognized that all three factors needed to be increased in some way; however, the group had insufficient time to explore specific ways of accomplishing this goal.

There was not enough time to devise other implementing strategies (e.g., to increase research/technology, to improve the quality of personnel preparation programs, to combat the generic trend, and to resolve the problems related to services in rural areas of the nation). It was hoped that other groups or additional study of the problems would be able to expand those areas more fully.

Chapter 7

VISIONS OF THE FUTURE

Dr. Natalie Barraga, Professor Emerita

University of Texas at Austin

Today you have heard "visions of the future" in technology, families, education, and future populations of persons with low vision. There are many ideas you can think about, many research projects you can consider, and a variety of practices you can implement on your own. Just now you have heard summaries of your own planning groups—what you think might be possible, what we need to do to make things happen, and how we might bring all of these things about.

But I have some dreams too, so when we gather again, perhaps we will be reflecting upon horizons far beyond the University of Texas, the state of Texas, and even the United States. With our capacity to reach countries across the oceans in a matter of hours, other planets in a day or so, and to communicate with colleagues anywhere in minutes, we are not bound to a small area or to service only a small group of persons with low vision. Through advances in technology, the world has become your classroom, and I challenge you to spread your wings.

To set the stage for your flight into the world beyond, let me reflect upon some of the happenings in that world in the last 25 years.

Did you know that . . .

- The first papers presented to the International Council for Education of the Visually Handicapped (ICEVH) on low vision were entitled "Border-liners—Problems of the Visually Handicapped between the Blind and Partially Sighted." This was in Madrid, Spain, the same time that the organization changed its name from International Council for Education of Blind Youth (ICEBY).

- At this same conference in 1972, three resolutions dealing with low vision were passed:

    1. ICEVH should seek to educate the public and give greater attention to those who may be needlessly considered blind when they have vision which may be utilized effectively.

    2. A functional definition of blindness was recommended and should be based on a total team evaluation and not on medical acuity alone.

    3. Children with residual vision are capable of responding to organized training and to function more efficiently; all teaching and medical disciplines should accept this in the assessment of visually handicapped children. ICEVH urges the extension of knowledge and

material for visual stimulation, and circulation of flexible and imaginative programs for children with usable vision.

- A school for the blind in England in 1964, requested assessment of their children for planning a program to teach them to use their vision, and to acquire appropriate visual materials.

- In 1974, the Australian and New Zealand Conference for Educators of the Visually Handicapped (ANZEVH) devoted their entire conference to all aspects of low vision, including optical aids and mobility, as well as assessment and learning programs for children.

- In 1974, the first three-day course on low vision for teachers in Brazil resulted in the translation of low vision material into Portuguese.

- The Research Institute in Birmingham, England, held a week-long seminar on low vision for teachers in residential schools for the blind in 1975.

- In 1976, the American Academy of Ophthalmology and the International Academy of Ophthalmology recommended that the World Health Organization (WHO) adopt new definitions of "blind" and "low vision" so that persons with vision were no longer called blind.

- By 1977, articles and materials on low vision had been translated into six different languages, and by 1989 into more than a dozen other languages.

- A conference on research in low vision was held in Uppsala, Sweden, in 1978 with papers invited from the University of Texas.

- Dr. Barraga and Dr. Corn led workshops in low vision and optical aids for all teachers of visually handicapped in Israel in 1971.

- In the last 10 years, members of the vision faculty of the University of Texas, along with graduates of the program in leadership positions, have conducted short courses, presented series of papers, and/or consulted with professional colleagues in Argentina, Brazil, China, Colombia, Ecuador, France, Germany, Guatemala, Holland, India, Malaysia, New Zealand, Panama, Scotland, Spain, Sri Lanka, Switzerland, and Taiwan.

- At ICEVH in 1987, an entire day was devoted to 12 workshop sessions on low vision involving former students and faculty from the University of Texas as leaders.

- Students have come to study in the vision program at the University of Texas from Australia, Chile, Finland, Germany, Kenya, Norway, and Sweden in the last 15 years.

- Since 1974, low vision clinics have been established in at least 10 different countries.

These events tell you that there aren't too may places in the world that have not heard of the University of Texas at Austin, especially on the topic of low vision. Need you ask what some of the challenges for the future may be considered paramount? For starters, here are just a few:

Expand your communication linkages with your colleagues in the state, the nation and around the world. In this age of fax machines and telecommunications, that is not as difficult as it might seem.

Make stronger communication efforts with colleagues in other disciplines so that the best of all knowledge can be applied to persons with low vision. Other professionals need to know what we can offer them in practical knowledge, and we need their expertise in new information about children and youth.

Keep records of your work, write up your experiences and studies, and share them at conferences and in journal articles. Perhaps in the next 25 years, you will document and share so much that we won't keep reinventing the wheel because we didn't know that someone else had already done it.

Think big, nationally and internationally. Learn and share with teachers around the world. We are all working for the same children, just in different ways and in a variety of cultural and political settings. The objectives and the process are the same and can be adapted to any situation everywhere in the world.

Join international organizations and read journals from other countries. Become actively involved with professionals through letters, contacts when traveling, presentations, and attendance at conferences. Start now to save your pennies for ICEVH in Singapore in 1992. I'll see you there!

Volunteer in time and energy for teaching short courses or conducting workshops in developing countries in return for expenses. Such experiences can teach you far more than any college course.

Find ways to determine how to make sure that multihandicapped children develop and use all of their vision to promote development and raise their quality of life.

Through such a worldwide approach, the same level of interest and learning about low vision persons and their needs can be broadened and maintained into the next century. If so, the programs and resources may continue to increase. The crucial responsibility is to see that low vision disciplines are able to double the rate of progress made in the last 25 years throughout the next 25 years, so that the high percentage of individuals with low vision will, at last, be seen as individuals with needs and services never before provided in all parts of the world. We are on the way, but we are not yet there.

When we gather here in 2014 to celebrate the 50th anniversary of the vision program, I hope to hear scintillating reports of your exploits in meeting these challenges. The stage is yours: Lights—camera—action.

PART TWO: FUTURES IN LOW VISION
RESEARCH PROJECT

INTO THE FUTURE

In two days, participants in the symposium had reached across 50 years—from 1964, when the Program to Prepare Teachers of the Visually Handicapped began at the University of Texas, to the year 2014, when a new wave of innovations and influences will alter the field. They had shared memories, renewed friendships, and rekindled the enthusiasm that drew them to the field of education for visually impaired children and youths.

To allow the ideas and goals to flicker out with the end of the symposium would seem a waste of resources. The two days had been filled with many memorable moments. But the event that provided a true link with the future was the Futures Session. The diversity of ideas about what the future will hold and the different ways in which the future can be shaped emphasized that the participants could have an impact on what will happen to people with low vision.

If a hundred conference participants could articulate their hopes and concerns for the future in a single afternoon, what would be the result if hundreds of other individuals involved in the field of low vision could also contribute their thoughts? What would be the similarities and differences in their views? Would they see themselves as influential in shaping the future? These questions motivated Drs. Bishop, Corn, and Erin to develop a study of the future of low vision that extended past June of 1989 and that reached beyond those who were connected with the University of Texas.

The force-field analysis used at the symposium formed the basis for a wide-ranging study of future thinking among those in the field of low vision. In the year following the symposium, a three-part study was conducted to investigate the predictions and influences that a group of respondents from many geographic areas with a variety of perspectives thought were important. In Part 2 of this monograph, the future moves out of the microcosm of Austin, Texas, and into the macrocosm of the world of low vision. The study that was conducted is reported in the following pages. The report includes a discussion of study methodology, a description of each phase of the project, and an examination of the results. Materials relating to study mailings, questionnaires, and responses appear in the appendixes. In addition, Chapters 11 and 12, authored by Dr. Kathleen M. Huebner and Dr. Virginia E. Bishop, respectively, offer two perspectives on the implications of the futures study.

Chapter 8

FUTURES PROJECT: PHASE 1

Virginia E. Bishop, Ph.D., Anne L. Corn, Ed.D., and Jane N. Erin, Ph.D.

University of Texas at Austin

INTRODUCTION

The future is no longer the private domain of psychics, seers, and soothsayers. It has become of vital interest to diverse groups in society. Politicians; economists; industrialists; and, lately, educators have discovered that some kind of forecasting is helpful in planning for the future. Moreover, corporations and governments have been using futurist techniques for some time. The RAND Corporation was originally created to assist the federal government in military forecasting, insurance companies and banks are studying trends, opinion researchers in marketing monitor changing attitudes of the public, and oil companies use scenario techniques for contingency planning. It is clear that the study of the future has become an essential tool in issues management, decision making, and planning.

All the approximately 150 techniques used in futures research have the same goal: to prepare for the future by anticipating changes in environments and in the needs of various populations. It is believed that such preparation will enable those who do so to manage and even direct the future. Forecasting can help determine where change is needed—what to facilitate and what to restrain. It can identify trends and alternatives. It can even extrapolate the future from an analysis of the past.

Forecasting should not be confused with prediction. The former projects what can happen, whereas the latter states what will happen. Forecasting includes the possibilities for issues management—the control of change. Futures research focuses on forecasting, emphasizing the systematic collection and analysis of data.

This project used force-field analysis—a futures research approach—because it seemed to be the best technique for issues management in the field of blindness and visual impairment and for using collective opinion to establish priorities and identify strategies. Investigators who apply this technique collect opinions about future events, examine the probability and impact of the events, and attempt to identify the factors or forces that may influence the occurrence (or nonoccurrence) of the events. Force-field analysis can be implemented within a few months and allows investigators to focus on a narrow topic.

It is hoped that the information accumulated and presented here will find its way to policymakers and planners in the field of visual impairment. Controlled change is possible only through foresight, and intentional issues management is a vital tool for a future-minded society.

PURPOSE

This study was conducted to identify issues and events that would influence the future of services for visually impaired people, to determine the likelihood of the occurrence and the degree of impact of these issues and events, to identify the desirability or undesirability of the identified events and issues, and to identify the strategies that would influence the occurrence of these events.

SUBJECTS

Potential respondents (*N* = 547) were selected from three sources: the *Directory of Agencies Serving the Visually Handicapped* (now the *Directory of Services for Blind and Visually Impaired Persons in the United States and Canada),* published by the American Foundation for the Blind (AFB), a list of parents obtained from the National Association for Parents of the Visually Impaired (NAPVI), and a list of graduates from the University of Texas Program to Prepare Teachers of the Visually Handicapped. Questionnaires were also sent to consumer organizations, such as the American Council of the Blind (ACB), Council of Citizens with Low Vision, Independent Visually Impaired Enterprises, National Alliance of Blind Students, National Association of Blind Teachers, and National Federation of the Blind (NFB) since there seemed to be no readily available mailing list of individuals; it was hoped that the organizations would make the questionnaires available to their members. In addition, a small list of international professionals was generated from the International Council for the Education of the Visually Handicapped (ICEVH); from selected attendees of recent conferences in Wurtzburg, Germany, and Edinburgh, Scotland; and from among the authors of articles in the January 1989 issue of the *Journal of Visual Impairment & Blindness* (which focused on worldwide services to visually impaired persons) (see Table 1; Tables 1-5 relating to the study can be found at the end of Chapter 10). In all cases, permission was granted to reproduce and circulate the survey materials, since the objective was to collect as many responses as possible.

Three rounds of questionnaires (corresponding to the three phases of the study) were mailed to the same persons and organizations, so the responses would be consistent and a consensus of opinion could be reached. The mailings were coded to track subgroups, but the anonymity of the respondents was maintained.

PROCEDURES: PHASE 1

The initial step of the project was to identify the issues or events to be studied. The vehicle for the identification phase was the low vision symposium at the University of Texas at Austin. Since the theme of the symposium was "Visions of the Future" and speakers had been asked to project their ideas 25 years into the future (to the year 2014), issues were defined by the four major areas addressed at the symposium: education, technology, the family, and the environment. Twenty-five event statements were generated from the symposium speakers' presentations. These event statements emerged from the issues raised by the speakers but were not necessarily statements with which each speaker would agree. The event statements became the focus of the first phase of the project.

Four of the event statements were discussed at the symposium, but because of time constraints, the full force-field analysis technique could not be completed there. This project represented a more thorough analysis of the event statements that was accomplished through a multiple mailing procedure, over a three-month period.

The first mailing was sent to the 547 potential respondents. Although the respondents were asked to identify their roles, so subgroups could be determined for data analysis, their anonymity was maintained to avoid any influence by colleagues or others. The respondents were first asked to state the likelihood that each event statement would occur by the year 2014, on a four-point Likert scale (from least likely to most likely), and then to estimate the impact of the event if it did occur (again, on a four-point Likert scale, from low impact to high impact). They were given two weeks to return questionnaires, which were coded to facilitate the tracking of the subgroups' responses (see Appendix A for the first mailing).

RESULTS

The response rate is reported for the entire set of 250 responses (although only 201 of them were received by the due date). A 46 percent response rate was noted for the full set of returned questionnaires, with rates exceeding 50 percent for 7 of the 11 subgroups—all three educator groups, the personnel preparation group, rehabilitation centers, parents, and support agencies (see Table 2). No subgroup had more than a 20 percent share of the responses, but 67 percent of the responses came from five groups: residential schools, public schools, personnel preparation programs, instructional materials centers and libraries, and rehabilitation centers. There were no responses from consumers.

Table 2 presents a summary of response data. It should be noted that in order to examine consensus within subgroups, it was arbitrarily established that at least one-third of the respondents had to agree.

Statements for further study were selected on the basis of highest impact–highest likelihood, a strong consensus on high impact–high likelihood, or the highest impact regardless of the likelihood. Twelve event statements were selected for continued study in Phase 2 of the project.

Data were examined to see if the respondents tended to agree among themselves within subgroups and between subgroups. (As already indicated, an arbitrary one-third consensus was used.) The personnel preparation respondents had the least amount of agreement. The highest agreement within subgroups was among the low vision center respondents and among parents, each group agreeing internally on nine items, six of which were the same in these two groups. These statements were as follows:

Item 1. An increased understanding of brain and neurological functioning as it relates to sight and seeing, has resulted in improved methods of teaching the visually impaired.

Item 8. Child care and early intervention programs for visually impaired children are required to have specially certified teachers.

Item 10. Increased prevalence among the aging population has resulted in greater acceptance of individuals with visual impairment.

Item 12. In spite of increasing numbers of minority children with visual impairments, the number of minority professionals in the field has decreased.

Item 14. Improved computer data base management has resulted in interagency (i.e., APH, Library of Congress, RFB, etc.) coordination and more effective tracking and programming for visually impaired children.

Item 23. Computers interpret brain waves, simulating visual experience; functional vision evaluations are no longer required, since professionals can now "view" what a child or adult is seeing.

Two other subgroups—the state-level vision consultants and the international professionals—also had internal consensus on five items each. Item 14 was the only common statement on which both subgroups agreed.

The subgroup of support agencies had an internal consensus on seven items; two of the items were the same as two items on which the state-level vision consultants agreed, and two items were consistent with the consensus among both the low vision centers and the international professionals. One item, Item 20, was consistent only with the consensus of the low vision centers:

Item 20. Due to high demand and low supply of teachers for the visually impaired, salary levels are considerably higher.

Several statements were listed in four or more subgroup consensus data. These were Items 8, 10, 14, and 6, which was as follows:

Item 6. Reductions in cost and size of low vision aids, along with added versatility, have permitted these aids to be programmed (computerized) to meet individualized needs, pathologies, and/or tasks.

An initial analysis of items was done for the 201 responses that were received by the due date, since the time line for the project required the use of these data in preparation for the second mailing. (A subsequent analysis of the entire set of 250 responses supported the conclusions drawn from the initial group of responses.)

A matrix was constructed to record the Likert-scale responses on the likelihood and impact of the event statements; only items receiving 30 or more votes were recorded on the matrix (see Table 3). (It was not useful to report these data by subgroups, since the numbers were too small and the opinions were diverse.)

Consensus of opinion within the subgroups was an interesting aspect of the data. The group of personnel preparation responses revealed the least amount of agreement.

Item 14 elicited a clear consensus (both within and between subgroups) about its likelihood and impact and appeared to be a hot issue among the respondents. Three other statements also were in this high-priority group: low vision aids were anticipated to become smaller, less costly, and more individualized (even programmable for unique needs, tasks, or pathologies). The increasing number of elderly visually impaired persons was believed to be an important factor in greater acceptance of *all* visually impaired people, and it was believed that an increase in the understanding of how children with low vision learn would enhance the teaching of visual efficiency.

A belief in the likelihood and impact of six event statements was also revealed, but the strength of the consensus was slightly less concentrated in one block of the analysis matrix. Adapted automatic bank-teller machines and other graphic displays were assumed to be "well on the way" and would be utilized, low vision services were believed to be headed toward coverage by health insurance, early childhood teachers who serve visually impaired children would need special certification, and an increased understanding of the neurological components of vision would improve teaching methods for visually impaired children. The statement that suggested future assessments of children with multiple handicaps would separate out the effects of a visual impairment elicited general agreement of its high impact and likelihood, but there was a sufficient lack of consensus to suggest that some people were not confident of the statement's likelihood. One statement that was thought to be highly likely and of high impact was that residential schools would increasingly serve only children with severe multiple handicaps. It could not be determined whether this was a desirable or undesirable outcome; therefore, the inclusion of this statement in the next questionnaire was assured.

One event statement elicited a "very unlikely" and "low impact" opinion, which indicated that few respondents thought teachers of visually impaired children would ever be private practitioners. Item 13, which stated that teachers would have less contact with parents because of "increased litigation and bureaucratic constraint" was not thought to be likely, but if it happened, it would certainly have an impact.

Item 9 (which stated that the increased political power of older visually impaired persons because of their increasing numbers would influence funding for health and vision services) was indecisive; although the opinions were toward likelihood and impact, the agreement was not strong enough and the diversity of opinions made it too weak an issue to pursue in the second questionnaire. Item 13, which was selected to replace it on the basis of the initial data analysis and concerned decreased contact with parents due to increased litigation and bureaucratic constraint, turned out to be a much more controversial item, and ended up in the third questionnaire.

Item 24 had an unusual opinion split. It stated that since disability labels would not exist (relative to education), disability-related assessment would no longer be required. There was almost universal agreement that this event was highly unlikely; however, the impact was almost evenly split between the lowest and the highest impact. Even an examination of voting by subgroup did not yield any reason for this split. Fortunately, this item went into the second questionnaire and ended up in the final questionnaire.

The remaining 11 statements, although not chosen for the second questionnaire, were still of interest. Four of them were related to technology (environmental simulators for orientation and mobility (O&M) instruction, miniaturized television cameras that could simulate vision, artificial vision systems, and computer simulations of visual experiences via the interpretation of brain waves). Two other statements were related to medicine and health care, and four more statements concerned the status of special education and education of visually impaired students. The final unchosen statement suggested that the field of visual impairment would retain its current status into the 21st century.

DISCUSSION

Three areas of concern will be discussed: the response rate, consensus among and within subgroups, and the event statements. Since the response rate was better than expected (nearly half the questionnaires were completed and returned), there were sufficient responses to draw some guarded conclusions. Although the number of responses in individual subgroups was too small to generalize the results, the total set of responses suggested some interesting conclusions.

It was unfortunate that no consumers responded to the questionnaire, since the event statements were especially relevant to them. It must be assumed that the consumer organizations to which the questionnaires were sent either did not have sufficient time to relay the questionnaires to their members or did not think that their constituents would care to respond. In either case, the result was that the people whose interest formed the central topic of investigation did not participate or express their opinions.

The high response rate suggests that the topics presented were of interest to the populations surveyed or that the method of research was novel to the respondents. A high level of interest could be expected from professionals in education and rehabilitation, but it was satisfying to note that quite a few ophthalmologists and optometrists, as well as individuals who work in libraries and in other professional capacities, completed the questionnaires. This finding suggests an increasing interest in cooperative programming—a long-anticipated practice in the field of visual impairment. The high response rate from parents suggested that these individuals are beginning to assume their rightful role in the educational-rehabilitation process.

With respect to the lack of agreement among personnel at colleges and universities, it may be speculated that the respondents in this group are unusually strong, creative, and independent personalities whose educational backgrounds and work settings vary considerably. Their independence and individuality may sometimes work against them as a group, since they seemed to disagree more than to agree on issues that may have an impact on personnel preparation and education of those with low vision.

Although it was reassuring to note the high level of agreement among several subgroups, there may be another subtle message in the consensus—that there is a fine line between conformity for conformity's sake and agreement because an item is in the best interest of those who receive services. It is hoped that the high consensus in these subgroups reflects thoughtful agreement, not "expected" opinion.

Twelve of the 13 statements that were not selected for the second questionnaire were dropped because there was a lack of agreement among the respondents. The thirteenth statement (Item 19) was dropped because of the ratings of low likelihood and low impact. Generally, the votes were too scattered to analyze. Apparently, these topics were either too imaginative (as in the technology-related items) or too controversial (national accreditation, teachers' salaries, lack of change or improvement in the field) and the opinions of the respondents were too widely diverse to achieve any kind of consensus.

Chapter 9

FUTURES PROJECT: PHASE 2

Virginia E. Bishop, Ph.D., Anne L. Corn, Ed.D., and Jane N. Erin, Ph.D.

University of Texas at Austin

Items for the study's second questionnaire were selected according to areas of interest on the matrix. Seven statements were selected from the highest likelihood–highest impact section of the matrix. Then the remaining blocks in the lower-right quadrant of the matrix (high likelihood–high impact) were examined, and an additional two items of high consensus (40 or more votes) were added. Finally, the highest impact (regardless of likelihood) column was examined, and three more items were selected. A total of 12 event statements were included in the second questionnaire, for which the respondents were asked to perform three operations for each statement: (1) determine the desirability or undesirability of the event if it were to occur; (2) list the forces that may cause the event to occur (facilitators) or that may keep it from occurring (restrainers); and (3) weight the forces, so that the total (facilitators and restrainers) equals 10 (see Appendix B for the second mailing).

The data analysis consisted of first determining the desirability or undesirability of each event statement and then examining the weights of the restraining or facilitating forces. If there was an obvious consistency between the desirability and the predominating (more heavily weighted) force, the item was discarded. It was assumed that the forces would bring about the anticipated outcome, with no intervention needed.

An event statement was included in the final questionnaire if it met any of the following conditions:

1. There was dissonance between desirability and forces (i.e., stronger restrainers for a desirable event or stronger facilitators for an undesirable event; any strength of dissonance was accepted).

2. Restrainers or facilitators were less than the established criteria of plus or minus 50.

3. There was a marked split of opinion about the desirability of the event.

One item met the first criterion, four items met the second criterion, and one item met the third criterion. A total of five items were included in the final questionnaire because one item met the criteria for both dissonance and split opinion.

RESULTS

The response rate for Phase 2 was less than half of the response rate for Phase 1: A total of 112 questionnaires were returned (out of 547 sent). About one-fifth of the respondents represented rehabilitation centers and offices, and 27 percent represented educators.

The overall response rate for all subgroups combined was 21 percent; the subgroup with the highest response rate was the personnel preparation programs group (38 percent), with low vision centers having the lowest rate of response (10 percent).

When the 12 statements were examined for their desirability and force weight, it was found that the respondents considered 9 to be desirable and 3 to be undesirable. Two items were unanimous opinions. Because not all the questionnaires contained complete data, some votes were missing.

The force weight was tallied separately for facilitating and restraining forces for each statement and then the difference between force weights was computed for each statement. If the difference was a positive number, it indicated a stronger facilitating force for that event, whereas if it was a negative number, it revealed a stronger restraining force. Differences of greater than 50 were speculated to be sufficient to cause an event to move in the direction of the more powerful force (restraining or facilitating).

In selecting items to be used in the final questionnaire, the investigators first used the criterion of dissonance. One statement—Item 8—met this criterion. That is, the respondents thought that the use of the residential school only for students with severe multiple handicaps was an undesirable outcome, but the facilitating forces were considerably stronger than were the restrainers. This item also had a split opinion about its desirability; 36 respondents thought it was desirable, and 63 thought it was undesirable.

Four statements had forces that may be too weak to ensure the outcome preferred by the respondents. Two items—6 (which referred to reduced contact with families due to litigation and bureaucratic constraints) and 11 (which suggested that individual assessments may no longer be required because disability labels had disappeared)—had weak restraining forces. Two statements—1 (which implied improved methods for teaching visually impaired children because of an increased understanding of brain and neurological function) and 4 (which specified that early childhood programs serving visually impaired children would require specially certified teachers)—had weak facilitators. Since items 1 and 6 had unanimous opinions about desirability, the weak forces were areas of concern and ensured the statements' positions in the final questionnaire.

When the forces for each statement were examined, they often reflected similar thoughts from a number of respondents. Therefore, to facilitate reporting, forces were consolidated into topical areas and listed for each event statement. The selected event statements are listed in Table 4; the facilitators and restrainers for each event statement are presented in Appendix C.

DISCUSSION

The study's second questionnaire was obviously more difficult and time consuming to complete than was the first; however, over a hundred respondents took the time to do so. The answers were generally thoughtful and relevant. Some issues elicited many similar answers (such as "more funding," "more research," "better teacher preparation," and "advocacy"), whereas others required more creative thinking. It was not the purpose of this project to pursue all questions. Only the items that met the criteria for further examination were selected for the final questionnaire. As was anticipated, there were a number of new respondents to this questionnaire, in addition to some who had also completed the first survey. Forty-four new individuals responded, along with 68 people who had completed the original survey.

Two statements elicited unanimous opinions about their desirability. That is, the respondents were extremely confident that breakthroughs in neurological research would have an impact on teaching methods for visually impaired children and that lessened contact between teachers and families was not a desirable outcome. The unanimity of these two opinions was not supported by the force weights, however. Although a greater understanding of brain function was thought to be highly desirable, there seemed to be a number of negative forces that could severely affect the outcome. The respondents also lacked some confidence in the forces that would prevent a widening gap between teachers and families. Because of the relatively weak forces at work for these two events, they were selected for further study in the third questionnaire.

Six statements were believed to be highly desirable, but the respondents' opinions were not totally unanimous. Four of these had forces that appeared to be strong enough to bring the events to fruition (more accessible bank-teller machines and other graphic displays, programmable low vision devices, greater acceptance of individuals with visual impairment because of an increasing number of elderly people with low vision, and a central computer data base to coordinate agency services and track programming). The remaining two statements had weaker facilitating forces, but still appeared to be viable possibilities in the future (insurance coverage for low vision services and vision rehabilitation specialists, and more sophisticated assessments that would separate the effects of a visual impairment for children with multiple handicaps).

Two event statements had a majority opinion of their desirability, but had a slightly higher level of disagreement than the other statements. The first, regarding specially certified teachers for young visually impaired children, was deemed desirable, but the opinion was certainly not unanimous. Moreover, the strength of forces required to achieve the event was weak. (This event was studied further in the final questionnaire.) The second, concerning increasing knowledge about how children with low vision learn, had weaker forces, but the forces were strong enough to instill confidence in the probability of the event's occurrence.

Statement 11, related to the disappearance of disability labels in education, was thought to be undesirable, but there was some disagreement among respondents. Most respondents did not believe that disability labels would disappear, since their disappearance would eliminate the disability-related assessments that are now required. The restraining forces were appropriately stronger, but perhaps not as strong as they could be. Therefore, this statement was examined further in the final questionnaire.

The final event statement concerned the role of residential schools. Although the designation of these schools only for children with severe multiple handicaps was noted as undesirable by 63 persons, over a third of the respondents thought that this role was appropriate. Facilitating forces outweighed restraining forces, which made the event statement a real possibility. Because of the split vote on the desirability of this event statement and the dissonance between forces and desirability, this event was included in the third questionnaire.

In summary, in Phase 2 the desirability, probable forces, and force weight of 12 event statements were studied. When there was a match between desirability and force weight, the item was discarded; the respondents apparently thought that the forces would bring about the predicted outcome with no interference. Statements whose forces were deemed too weak to cause the desired results or statements whose desirability and forces disagreed were chosen for the final questionnaire. Five event statements qualified.

Chapter 10

FUTURES PROJECT: PHASE 3

Virginia E. Bishop, Ph.D., Anne L. Corn, Ed.D., and Jane N. Erin, Ph.D.

University of Texas at Austin

Data from Phase 2 of the study were analyzed on the basis of 100 returns received by the due date (although the final data included 112 responses). Of the five event statements selected for further study in Phase 3, four had weak forces that placed the desired outcomes at risk and one appeared to generate considerable controversy. The goal of Phase 3 was to elicit strategies to strengthen the forces of four of the events and to probe in more depth the opinions of the respondents on the controversial statement (see Appendix D for the third mailing).

Data were tallied by content and frequency. Then, each event statement was examined to see which forces were chosen by most of the respondents and to identify the respondents' suggestions of strategies for implementation. For the first four event statements, forces that were selected 10 or more times (by approximately 10 percent of the respondents) were examined more closely. Strategies were analyzed for their similarity and were listed by general content.

For the last event statement, all forces were examined and strategies were analyzed for similarities. The event statements were listed to reveal their most-selected forces and the common strategies that were suggested.

RESULTS

The overall response rate for Phase 3 (19.6 percent) was nearly the same as for Phase 2 (20.5 percent). Residential school personnel made up nearly one-fifth of the respondents, with teacher educators and rehabilitation centers each contributing slightly less than one-fifth of the returns. Teacher-educators had the highest within-subgroup response rate (40 percent), followed by residential school personnel (33 percent), public school personnel (28 percent), state-level vision consultants (28 percent), and support agencies (21 percent). Consumers again did not respond (see Table 2).

The five event statements, along with the strategies for facilitation and restraint, are described next. Only those strategies that were suggested by more than 10 percent of the respondents are reported here. (An entire listing of strategies is available from the editors of this report.)

Event 1: An increased understanding of brain and neurological functioning as it relates to sight and seeing, has resulted in improved methods of teaching the visually impaired. This event was considered to be desirable by *all* the respondents in Phase 2. The facilitating forces (the forces that could cause the event to occur) were thought to be weak, however, and the forces that might impede the event were believed to be stronger than they should be. Thus, the event needed some additional help if it was to occur; the restraining forces would have to be eliminated, and the facilitating forces would have to be strengthened. The following forces were selected for designing strategies by at least 10 percent of the respondents:

Facilitators

1. Closer cooperation between medicine and education.

2. Cooperative research between medicine and education.

3. Translation of research into teaching strategies.

4. More comprehensive teacher preparation, including a course in neuroanatomy.

5. In-service training to update teacher skills.

Restrainers

1. Rigidity of medical thinking regarding education.

2. Lack of funding for research.

3. Poor communication of research findings (i.e., lag time between research and practice).

4. Lack of cooperation between education and medicine.

5. Shortage of VH teachers [teachers of visually impaired students].

Event 2: Due to increased litigation and bureaucratic constraint, teachers have less contact with families during the educational program planning process. This event was considered to be undesirable by *all* the respondents in Phase 2, but the restraining forces (the forces that could keep it from happening) were not seen as strong enough to ensure that it would not occur. If this event is to be prevented from happening, the restrainers must be stronger, and the facilitators must be weakened or neutralized.

Facilitators

1. Time constraints because of heavy caseloads.

2. Lack of training in how to work with parents.

3. IEP [Individualized Education Program] process views parent role as token participation becomes confrontational.

Restrainers

1. Parent awareness of rights.

2. Increase in parent-teacher partnership.

3. Training in consultation methods for teachers.

4. Extra pay for after-hours consultation with parents.

5. Parent opinions encouraged, respected, and valued (an additional related and often chosen restraining force).

6. Teachers trained to work with parents.

Event 3: Child care and early intervention programs for visually impaired children are required to have specially certified teachers. This event was considered to be desirable by 88 percent of the respondents but it was not considered likely to occur. Restraining forces were believed to be strong enough to prevent the event from happening. If the desired outcome is to be achieved, the facilitating forces need to be considerably stronger, and the restraining forces should be eliminated or at least neutralized. The following forces were selected for designing strategies by at least 10 percent of the respondents.

Facilitators	*Restrainers*
1. Parent pressure-advocacy.	1. Lack of personnel (teachers).
2. National emphasis on early intervention.	2. Services unavailable in rural areas.
3. Greater understanding of the impact of visual impairment on early development.	3. Generic special education trend.
4. Stipends-monetary encouragement for additional training (e.g., VH certification [certification in visual impairment] plus early childhood, or vice versa).	4. Lack of teacher preparation programs.

Additional related and often chosen forces:

5. Professional pressure (e.g., AER [Association for Education and Rehabilitation of the Blind and Visually Impaired]).	5. Insensitivity to the needs of young visually impaired children.

Event 4: Disability labels no longer exist relative to education; therefore, individualized assessment of specific disabilities is no longer required. This event was considered to be undesirable by 86 percent of the respondents. The restraining forces were stronger than the facilitating forces, but the difference was not enough to be confident of the outcome. If the event is to be prevented with any degree of certainty, the restraining forces will have to be strengthened and the facilitating forces will have to be weakened or neutralized. The following forces were selected for designing strategies by at least 10 percent of the respondents:

Facilitators

1. Generic trend.

2. All teachers trained in all exceptionalities.

Restrainers

1. Advocacy for individualization.

2. Improved teacher preparation, especially in assessment.

3. Required practicum in assessment for VH teachers [of visually impaired students].

4. Strict implementation of the laws requiring assessment.

5. Joint efforts between teachers and parents to maintain individual assessments.

6. Legislative awareness of the need for specialized teaching methods.

Additional related and often-chosen forces:

1. Denial of disability on the part of parents.

2. Shortage of special teachers.

3. VH [visually handicapped] students recognized as needing special disability-related assessment.

Event 5: State schools and other institutions for the visually impaired serve only the most severely involved multiply handicapped children. This event was highly controversial in Phase 2 (64 percent of the respondents thought it would be an undesirable outcome, but 36 percent believed it would be desirable). The forces were strongly weighted in the direction of the event's occurrence. Therefore, if the event is to be prevented, the facilitators will have to be weakened or neutralized and the restrainers will have to be strengthened considerably. Since only 21 respondents addressed the facilitators, and only five addressed them directly, it was determined that the opinion was in favor of the restrainers) (78 respondents addressed the restrainers).

Most reasons given for keeping residential schools only for visually impaired children with the severest multiple handicaps were vaguely worded ("equity in a normalized setting," "collaborative programs in communities," "low vision evaluations will maximize visual potential"), but some statements actually negated the entire concept of a residential school ("close all residential schools" or "eliminate all state schools that segregate on the basis of disability"). No educators (residential school personnel, public school personnel, or state-level vision consultants) thought that residential schools should be only for visually impaired children with the severest multiple handicaps. The advocates of this view were among teacher-educators (5), rehabilitation centers (5), instructional materials centers and libraries (4), low vision centers (3), support agencies (2), and international professionals (2). The predominant opinion was that residential schools should be retained, but that their role and function need to be examined. The following forces were selected for designing strategies by at least 10 percent of the respondents:

Facilitators

1. Public schools unwilling to serve multiply handicapped children.

2. Deinstitutional movement.

3. Expanded public school programs serving a wider range of disabilities.

4. Rigid admission and dismissal procedures discourage short-term placement.

Restrainers

1. Short-term services for "normal" or moderately visually handicapped children available in the state school.

2. Recognizing when mainstreaming is appropriate and when it is not appropriate.

3. Full continuum required.

4. Broader interpretation of LRE [least-restrictive environment].

5. Expanded role of state school to include outreach services, evaluation, resource center.

6. Failures in mainstreaming.

7. Shortages of teachers in rural areas.

8. Focus on short-term placement, with goal of returning to home school.

9. Openness to MAP [most appropriate placement].

10. Sense of partnership between state schools and public schools in educating visually handicapped children.

11. Clearer articulation of role of the residential school.

DISCUSSION

Responses for Phase 3 required specific, concrete strategies for action. In some cases, these ideas were general ("promote," "lobby," "improve"), but most were articulate and straightforward. Both humor and strong feelings were expressed in the responses (for example, "Have Geraldo visit an early childhood class" and "Quit fighting!" written in inch-high capital letters). It was apparent that those who responded to Phase 3 had something to say and took the time to say it.

Event 1

The first statement (related to neurological function and vision) revealed an interest in the relationships between research and practice. Many respondents suggested strategies for increasing working relationships between the medical profession and educators. Although the statement referred to neurological function, the respondents appeared to include ophthalmologists among the "medical personnel." The need for educators to have access to and understand medical research was recognized, and a strong majority favored additional course work in neuroanatomy in teacher preparation programs. On the basis of the large number of responses that suggested increased cooperation between medicine and education, there appears to be a need to open the channels of communication between these two disciplines. The need to understand research suggests that some concrete action should be taken as soon as possible. Funding of research elicited few concrete strategies. "Campaigns," priorities," and "lobbying" were essential elements, but no "how to" or "who" materialized.

Strategies to end the shortage of teachers resurfaced in strategies for other statements. Recruitment remains a problem, and monetary incentives continue to be thought of as solutions. One creative solution was the creation of a "Peace Corps" of volunteers to get teachers to visually impaired children in areas where they are needed. The shortage of teachers is of great concern and will be addressed further in analyses of other statements.

In-service training was a concern that elicited a number of strategies, ranging from "packages" developed by the Association for Education and Rehabilitation of the Blind and Visually Impaired (AER) or by the Division for the Visually Handicapped of the Council for Exceptional Children (DVH) to specific-topic self-instruction modules. The responsibility for sponsorship ranged from teacher preparation programs and departments of education to a "network of key organizers." Again, this topic will be addressed further in discussions of other statements.

Event 2

The second statement (related to contact with the family) elicited strong feelings of commitment to the parent-teacher relationship. It was clear that the respondents thought that parents are critical factors in the educational process; however, it was also evident that the relationship could be strengthened. A number of strategies were related to learning how to communicate more effectively with parents and how to resolve conflicts. Administrators were included in the group of educators who needed to improve these skills, and several suggestions regarded in-service training for administrators as essential. Training in how to work with parents could be provided both at the preservice and in-service levels. Parents themselves were included in the strategies (such as joint in-service courses for parents and teachers, the active solicitation of parents' opinions, and inviting parents to speak at teacher preparation courses at universities).

The role of parents in the Individualized Education Program (IEP) process was perceived as critical, and it was realized that this role was often not as it should be. Again, administrators were targeted for some training in this area. The consensus seemed to be that parents should be encouraged to participate more actively in the IEP process, even if it means that professionals must abide by parents' wishes for their children's placement. Clearly, this problem needs to be addressed if the desired outcome of cooperative planning is to be achieved (and the threats of litigation are to be minimized).

The problem of when there is time to meet with parents was addressed from both a monetary and an administrative viewpoint. If contact with parents is to be at times other than during the work day, the consensus of opinion was that it should be reimbursed.

An alternate solution is to allow flexible work hours, so that parents can be seen when they are most available (late afternoon, evenings, and Saturdays). Decreasing caseloads will work only if there are enough teachers; therefore, until the shortage of teachers is alleviated, more creative (and possibly financially rewarding) solutions will have to be utilized to increase teachers' time with parents.

Event 3

The third statement concerned early intervention services for visually impaired children by certified teachers of the visually impaired. Two major issues emerged from the strategies: the impact of a visual impairment on early development (and the resulting urgent need for early intervention) and the appropriateness of the service providers. It was generally agreed that the general public (including early childhood specialists) is not aware of the effects of visual impairment on early development and that both public awareness programs and preservice-in-service training for early childhood personnel are needed; early childhood teachers need information on visual impairment, and teachers of the visually impaired need information about early childhood development. The suggested public awareness strategies ranged from public service announcements to an on-site visit by television commentator Geraldo Rivera with an early childhood class of visually impaired children.

Parental involvement was highlighted in some of the strategies, both collectively (through NAPVI) and individually. It was recognized that parents are "the bottom line," particularly in early childhood programs. It is parents who have the power to demand and make changes. Perhaps the wisest strategy would be to teach parents how to advocate effectively and then to unleash the potential power of their collective voice.

Several other issues regarding this event emerged as well: incentives for additional training, strategies for the delivery of services in rural areas, and coping with the trend toward generic special education. The respondents were almost unanimous in their opinion that some kind of monetary encouragement would be necessary for teachers to get additional training (whether in the area of early childhood or visual impairment). P.L. 99-457 was mentioned as a source of training funds; however, this law does not provide for personnel preparation (it refers back to regulations in P.L. 94-142 that cover personnel preparation). Monetary incentives will have to be built into grants or come from state-local budgets.

Several intriguing strategies were suggested for delivering services in rural areas, including a "Peace Corps" of volunteers and the use of trained or supervised aides, mobile units, and outreach services from residential schools. Since the shortage of teachers is a limiting factor, a creative solution will certainly be appropriate.

Event 4

The fourth statement was related to the possible elimination of disability labels and their accompanying disability-related assessments. Because the elimination of labels was perceived to be linked to the trend toward generic special education, a number of strategies concerned this trend. The common theme of these strategies was proving that a visual impairment causes unique problems in learning. Again, the suggestions ranged from disputing the generic special education philosophy to accepting it with exceptions (i.e., not including visually impaired children in the generic population). It was apparent that the respondents believed that this trend will not abate and that it must be dealt with. Lobbying (making the public, especially legislators, aware of the uniqueness of visual impairments) seemed to be the strategy of consensus.

The problem of appropriate assessments by trained evaluators had two facets: maintaining the availability of disability-related assessments and making well-trained evaluators available. Presently, P.L. 94-142 and most state laws *require* such special assessments for visually impaired children, but the respondents must have perceived that the requirement would be in danger of being eliminated if disability labels disappeared. Thus many strategies for keeping legislators and other policymakers aware of people with visual impairments were suggested.

The problem of having qualified evaluators to do the assessments emerged as a separate issue. There seemed to be a general agreement that evaluators (whether teachers of the visually impaired or psychologists-diagnosticians) are not well prepared to do the job. A number of strategies were suggested to remedy this problem. Both preservice and in-service courses (for teachers of the visually impaired) in assessment techniques were mentioned by a number of respondents, and a practicum was a condition of both types of training. It was not specified what types of assessment were in question (psychological; functional vision; or disability skills, such as O&M or braille) but it was recommended that psychologists-diagnosticians should participate in the recommended training. Perhaps the implication is that *all* types of evaluators of visually impaired children need more training and that some of the training may be cooperative.

The shortage of teachers was also an issue in this statement, and the strategies were similar to those offered in the other statements. Increased pay and decreased paperwork were suggested as incentives for recruiting teachers, and a job-placement strategy was mentioned as a way of using available talent most efficiently.

An interesting force emerged as a factor in the disappearance-of-labels issue. Parents' denial of their children's disability was addressed by a number of strategies. The respondents thought that teachers of the visually impaired often need to act as counselors (and may require special training to do so) and that parents often need counseling. It may be essential to help parents go through the grief process to reach the state of acceptance. As one respondent stated, parents need to learn to "cherish" the accomplishments of their visually impaired children without "ignoring" (or denying) their needs and available services. If teachers of the visually impaired take on the additional responsibility of counseling, they will first have to gain the skills to do so.

Event 5

The role of residential schools generated more interest than any other issue. The proponents of using residential schools only for visually impaired children with severe multiple handicaps did not address the facilitating forces directly enough to strengthen them, and their alternate statements were either vague ("more money for education"); equivocal ("adopt a departmental policy of having only the severely multiply handicapped in residential schools but allow options if local areas can't serve the visually impaired"); or strongly biased ("residential schools should not serve other visually impaired students because of overprotectiveness and cloistering"). It was difficult to sift any real strategies from these statements.

The predominant opinion seemed to be that the residential school not only fulfills a position on the continuum, but has the potential to make a positive contribution to the education of visually impaired children in general. Strategies fell into three broad categories (not counting the general statements): modification of the residential school, concerns with mainstreaming, and issues relevant to the least restrictive environment (LRE) and the most appropriate placement (MAP). The strategies related to mainstreaming were few, since it seems to be viewed as a mandate. The emphasis seemed to be on making sure that mainstreaming is working and to alleviate mainstreaming failures with alternative programming. The residential school was viewed as one such alternative.

The major concern was the interpretation of LRE and MAP (an issue that is now being reviewed at the federal level). A plea for an "open approach to MAP" and a broader interpretation of LRE seemed to be reflected in the proposed redefinition of LRE as the "most conducive environment."

An important issue that emerged from the strategies for this statement was the changing role of the residential school. The issue of visually impaired children with severe multiple handicaps did not surface, and it must be assumed that the majority of the respondents saw the residential school as an appropriate educational placement for these children. The important finding in this study, however, is that most respondents believed that the residential school has the potential for making a greater contribution to the educational arena. Among the support roles noted were short-term (less than a year) intensive training in compensatory skills (such as braille and O&M), summer programs for home-school credit in a variety of areas (including computers, daily living skills, O&M, and homemaking), the preparation of visually impaired students for mainstreaming (and a commitment to that end), outreach instruction and consultation, assessment and evaluation, model programs for observation, resource centers (for lending equipment and for itinerant teachers), on-site consultation, workshops and in-service courses, research centers, teacher education, and transitional planning. Moreover, one respondent even suggested that the residential school should establish regional centers throughout the state (it was presumed that the respondent was from a large state). As one respondent stated, there must be "better attempts to understand the *needs* of visually impaired students" and to base placements-services on needs, rather than on their availability. Instructional programs should be available at all levels of the continuum, and preferably in or near home schools. The reality, however, is that this ideal situation does not exist, and the best use must be made of available money and personnel. To quote another respondent, "residential schools and public schools should not be a threat to each other"; they should be simply choices on a mandated continuum.

SUMMARY AND CONCLUSIONS

At the completion of the study, a summary of response data was made. Since the subgroups had been tracked across all three phases of the study, it was a simple task to determine how many had responded to one, two, or all three phases (see Table 5). Although residential school personnel represented the highest number of respondents, they were followed closely by teacher-educators and staff of rehabilitation centers. It was apparent that many respondents moved in or out of the study as it progressed; only 38 people answered all three questionnaires. Staff members of rehabilitation centers provided about one-fourth of these continued responses.

Response rates could also be compared for the three mailings (see Table 2). The high rate for the first questionnaire was probably due to its simplicity; however, an almost equal rate for the second and third questionnaires suggested a commitment to the goals of the project by at least one-fifth of the people who were contacted. The highest within-subgroup response rate across the three mailings was the teacher-educator group. Consumers did not reply to any of the questionnaires.

In examining the content of items as they were deleted from each phase of the study, the investigator found that an interesting pattern emerged. Of the six original statements that referred to some aspect of low vision (as opposed to visual impairment), two were dropped from Phase 1 and the other four were lost in Phase 2. Of the six original statements related to technology, four were deleted in Phase 1 and two disappeared during Phase 2. The final five statements did not refer to low vision or to technology. The absence of these two topics in the final five statements may reflect that they are still not firmly established in the minds of people in the field of visual impairment. If this is the case, it is a cause for concern. Although current attitudes seem to favor the *use* of available vision (functional vision), rather than the conservation of vision (as was common in the 1950s), there is still much room for growth in thinking. This may be an area for further study, and it is certainly a topic for continued emphasis.

The broad concerns that were targeted by the respondents in this study seemed to be grouped into five areas: the trend toward generic special education, with its threat of ending categorical programs and funding; appropriate services for young visually impaired children; the role of parents in the educational process; the shortage of teachers, with the accompanying need to utilize the residential school in new and innovative ways; and the recognition that brain research may change our way of understanding how learning takes place. In all cases, the topics appear to reflect fears of diminishing control. Generic special education minimizes the effects of disabilities and reduces the role of specialists; responsibilities for educating young visually impaired children have suddenly fallen into untrained hands; parents are being encouraged to become more informed and to participate in decision making—a threat to the traditional position of power vested in "experts" in education; the shortage of teachers is forcing a reevaluation of the content and method of teacher education and of service delivery models; and there is a real possibility that educational theory will be turned upside down with discoveries of how the brain works and how learning occurs. We service providers and educators may be feeling so threatened by events and forces that we perceive to be beyond our control that we may be stamping out sparks when we should be fighting a forest fire. The "smoke" may be obscuring some much more important issues: imaginative applications of technology, creative uses of existing resources, and the need to change essential definitions.

This is not to say that the concerns raised by this study are unimportant. In the minds of the respondents, they were critical issues, to be managed *now*. We may *need* to reexamine problems, devise solutions, and take action. This project should provide a number of strategies to be tried, and it is hoped that many of them will be successful. We need to dream big, strive for things as yet unknown, and work toward the best possible environment for the people we serve, both now and in the future. If *any* change is effected by the findings presented here, then the goal of the study will have been achieved. The investigator hopes that visually impaired citizens in the year 2014 will be able to look back and thank the respondents in this study for their foresight and their courage in making an effort to control the direction of the future.

LIMITATIONS OF THE STUDY

Opinion research is imprecise at best, and forecasting techniques suffer from some of the same shortcomings. In data analysis, the investigator must use his or her judgment in interpreting responses, must group answers subjectively for efficiency in reporting, and must draw conclusions based on small samples. The reader never gets to see the original responses and must rely on the knowledge and experience of the investigator in interpreting them. It must be assumed that the investigator has an objective goal in mind, has predetermined criteria for evaluating the data, and maintains a high level of integrity in conducting the study.

Another limitation that is unique to forecasting is the unavoidable loss of data as the process continues. This project began with 25 event statements and concluded with five. The first phase eliminated 13 statements not because they would not occur or were not interesting, but because not enough respondents reached agreement on their likelihood or impact. If all 547 persons had responded, the additional 297 responses might have achieved a greater total consensus, but these persons chose not to express their opinions. The data had to be analyzed on the basis of the 250 responses received. There is no way of knowing whether any deleted statements would have produced additional useful information.

During the second phase of this study, forces were identified. The investigator had to rely on the collective perceptions of the respondents (which may or may not have been complete, accurate, or properly weighted) and to assume that the responses were valid and accurately perceived. There is no way of determining whether all possible forces were identified or whether the weighing was accurate. Again, the investigator had to rely on the assumed relative expertise of the respondents.

Unknown and unexpected forces can arise that can disrupt even the most carefully described forecast. Although such changes were not anticipated by the respondents, the reader must accept their possibility as a flaw in futures forecasting.

In the use of force-field analysis, the determination of dissonance is reasonably straightforward, but the establishment of criteria to suggest the "strength" or "weakness" of different forces is subjective. This investigator attempted to be conservative in establishing criteria, but once they were set, she adhered to them strictly. The reader may notice that although two statements were close to but exceeded the criteria for selection, a strict interpretation of the criteria eliminated them from the final questionnaire. Such a loss of potential data is unavoidable in forecasting.

The final data analysis was force related but subjectively interpreted. Every response was recorded, but grouped topically for reporting purposes. The investigator made every attempt to retain the original content, but any deviation from the original wording carries with it the potential for some loss of data. The value of the information lies in its relationship to the force for which strategies are to be devised. However, it is hoped that the original objective of the study was still met.

Table 1

RESPONSES BY ROLES

Educators

    Residential Schools for the Blind... 67

    Public Schools.. 46

    State-Level Vision Consultants 18

Teacher Preparation Personnel.. 47

Rehabilitation Offices/Centers 96

Instructional Materials Centers/Libraries 72

Low Vision Centers.. 92

Parents (of visually impaired children) 27

*Support Agencies (AFB, APH, NAC, NAVH, NSPB, RFB, etc.)............................. 38

Consumers..7

International Professionals 37

_____

Total Potential Respondents 547

* Support agencies included the American Foundation for the Blind (AFB), American Printing House for the Blind (APH), National Accreditation Council for Agencies Serving the Blind and Visually Handicapped (NAC), National Association for Visually Handicapped (NAVH), National Society to Prevent Blindness (NSPB), and Recording for the Blind (RFB).

Table 2

SUMMARY OF RESPONSE DATA FOR THE PROJECT

		E-1*	E-2	E-3	T	1	R	L	P	C	S	W	TOTALS
PHASE ONE	No. Rec'd	37	25	11	28	28	49	21	14	0	22	15	250
	Row %	14.8	10.0	4.4	11.2	11.2	19.6	8.4	5.6	0.0	8.8	6.0	---
	Col. %	55.2	54.3	61.1	59.6	38.9	51.0	22.8	51.9	0.0	57.9	40.5	45.7
PHASE TWO	No. Rec'd	16	11	3	18	11	24	9	4	0	11	5	112
	Row %	14.3	9.8	2.7	16.1	9.8	21.4	8.0	3.6	0.0	9.8	4.5	---
	Col. %	23.9	23.9	16.7	38.3	15.3	25.0	9.8	14.8	0.0	28.9	13.5	20.5
PHASE THREE	No. Rec'd	21	13	5	19	11	18	5	1	0	8	6	107
	Row %	19.6	12.1	4.7	17.8	10.3	16.8	4.7	1.0	0.0	7.5	5.6	---
	Col. %	32.8	28.3	27.8	40.4	15.3	18.8	5.4	3.7	0.0	21.1	16.2	19.6
	No. Sent	67	46	18	47	72	96	92	27	7	38	37	547
		12.2	8.4	3.3	8.6	13.2	17.6	16.8	4.9	1.3	6.9	6.8	

* See Table 5 for a key to the abbreviations used.

Table 3

COMPOSITE OF DATA FROM PHASE ONE (BASED ON 102 RETURNS)

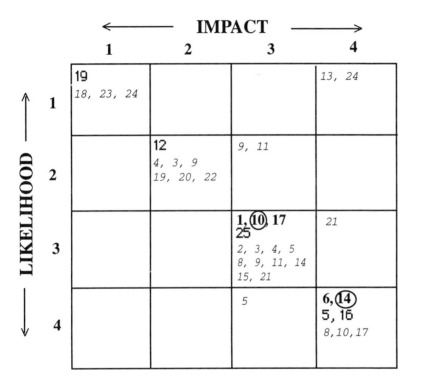

IMPACT →

	1	2	3	4
1	19 *18, 23, 24*			*13, 24*
2		12 *4, 3, 9* *19, 20, 22*	*9, 11*	
3			1,⑩, 17 25 *2, 3, 4, 5* *8, 9, 11, 14* *15, 21*	*21*
4			*5*	6,⑭ 5, 16 *8, 10, 17*

LIKELIHOOD

<u>No. Votes</u>
⑥⓪+ - 30%
50-59 - 25%
40-49 - 20%
30-39 - 15%

First Area of Interest: Highest Likelihood
Highest Impact
(i.e., 4-4)
14, 6, 5, 16, 8, 10, 17

Second Area of Interest: High Likelihood
High Impact
High Consensus
10, 1, 17, 25

Third Area of Interest: Highest Impact
Regardless of Likelihood
14, 6, 5, 16, 8, 10, 17, 13, 24, 21

Items Selected for Phase Two: 1, 5, 6, 8, 10, 13, 14, 16, 17, 21, 24, 25

Table 4

ANALYSIS OF
EVENT STATEMENTS SELECTED FOR PART TWO

EVENT	KEY	DESIR.		FORCES		DIF.
		Desir.	Undes.	Facil.	Restr.	
(1.) An increased understanding of brain and neurological functioning as it relates to sight and seeing, has resulted in improved methods of teaching the visually impaired.		107	0	494	466	+28
2. Automatic bank teller machines and other graphics displays have been converted to large print and/or speech output for greater access to the visually impaired.		104	3	574	342	+232
3. Reductions in cost and size of low vision aids, along with added versality, have permitted these aids to be "programmed" (computerized) to meet individual needs, pathologies and/or tasks.		96	8	499	396	+103
(4.) Child care and early intervention programs for visually impaired children are required to have specially certified teachers.		92	13	455	446	+9
5. Increased prevalence of low vision among the aging population, has resulted in greater acceptance of individuals with visual impairments.		99	5	514	315	+199
(6.) Due to increased litigation and bureaucratic constraint, teachers have less contact with families during the educational program planning process.		0	102	418	452	-34
7. Improved data base management has resulted in interagency (i.e., APH, Libarary of Congress, RFB, etc.) coordination and more effective tracking and programming for visually impaired children.		97	3	492	377	+115
(8.) State schools and other institutions for the visually impaired serve only the most severely involved multiply handicapped children.		36	63	488	396	+92
9. The knowledge of how children with low vision learn has been greatly expanded; therefore, teachers of the visually handicapped devote more service delivery time to teaching the use of available vision.		84	15	484	373	+111
10. Low vision and vision rehabilitation specialist services are covered by insurance and health care providers as a part of standard medical practice.		96	9	486	433	+53
(11.) Disability labels no longer exist relative to education; therefore, assessment of specific disabilities is no longer required.		14	87	402	447	-45
12. Sophisticated assessments allow the effects of vision to be distinguished from other disabilities present in the multiply handicapped child.		94	3	467	401	+66

KEY

- ▨ Original 4-4's
- ☐ Original 3-3's
- ☐ Original 4's

Original Item Selection Criteria From 1st Questionnaire

▦ High Likelihood High Impact

▦ High Impact

▦ High Impact Regardless of Likelihood

(For 3rd Questionnaire)
SELECTED ITEMS OF INTEREST

#1. Weak facilitating forces
#4. Weak facilitating forces
#6. Weak restraining forces
#8. Dissonance & split opinion
#11. Weak restraining forces

Table 5

SUMMARY OF RESPONSE DATA

	No. Responses			No. Responses in each combination							
Sub Group	Phase One	Phase Two	Phase Three	One Only	Two Only	Three Only	1 & 2	1 & 3	2 & 3	All Three	*Total
E-1	37	16	21	18	2	11	10	6	1	3	74
E-2	25	11	13	15	4	3	1	4	1	5	49
E-3	11	3	5	6	0	1	1	2	0	2	19
T	28	18	19	11	99	1	1	10	2	6	65
I	28	11	11	22	4	5	2	1	2	3	50
R	49	24	18	28	6	1	6	5	2	10	91
L	21	9	5	18	3	2	3	0	3	0	35
P	14	4	1	11	1	0	2	0	0	1	19
C	0	0	0	0	0	0	0	0	0	0	0
S	22	11	8	14	2	2	4	1	2	3	41
W	15	5	6	9	0	0	0	1	0	5	26
Totals	250	112	107	152	31	26	30	30	13	38	469

* Total number of responses, by subgroups, for entire project.

E-1 = Residential Schools   L = Low Vision Centers

E-2 = Public Schools   P = Parents

E-3 = State-Level Vision Consultants   C = Consumers

T   = Teacher Preparation Programs   S = Support Agencies

I   = Instructional Materials Centers and Libraries   W = International Professionals

R   = Rehabilitation Centers/Offices

Chapter 11

A CALL FOR INDIVIDUAL AND COLLABORATIVE EXPANSION OF THOUGHT AND RISK TAKING

Kathleen M. Huebner, Ph.D.

Director, National Program Associates
American Foundation for the Blind

People have always been intrigued by the unknown. However, throughout the ages, human beings' perceptions of our ability to affect the future have differed. Some believe that we will know the future when it arrives and before that we should not worry about it. Others believe that our task is not to foresee the future, but to enable it. Still others believe that the only way to predict the future is to have the ability to shape it. Today, many believe that even if we cannot control our destiny, we can influence both the immediate and distant future.

Some greet the unknown with zeal, whereas others think of it with great trepidation. Yet, more and more "we want to be in a position where we can at least start to forecast our own future" (Cetron & O'Toole, 1982, p. 3). As we enter the 21st century, we can look to authors, such as Toffler (1980) and Naisbitt (1984), whose books have served, in part, to prepare and comfort us about the future. In addition, novelists, including science fiction writers, and screenwriters have provided us with a plethora of futuristic fantasies or, some may think, true visions of impending realities, since much of yesterday's science fiction is, after all, today's reality.

In our lifetimes, we have seen what once were futuristic concepts come true. Many of us were born before television, frozen foods, credit cards, personal computers, fax machines, Patriot missiles, and space exploration. Most of us remember when a chip meant a piece of wood, hardware meant tools, and software was not a word. Did our predecessors envision Talking Books, VersaBraille, Kurzweil Reading Machines, and talking blood-glucose monitors? Did we foresee audiodescription services and Talking Newspapers? Yet, the creative among us recognized a need and met the challenge through invention and determination.

At this time in our field's history, a time of accelerated progress due largely to technological advancements, we do not have to be convinced of the potential for dramatic innovative change. Efforts from many fields of study will ultimately lead to the achievement of "equality of access and opportunity that will ensure freedom of choice" for individuals who are blind and visually impaired (American Foundation for the Blind, 1991).

Forecasting the future is not like playing a game of chance. It is a process that requires the "collection, analysis and synthesis of data" (Cetron & O'Toole, 1982, p. 4). Professional forecasting had its beginnings at the start of World War II. Today, nearly a dozen organizations in the United States do professional forecasting. The study described in the previous chapters presents clear examples of forecasting, stimulated by the symposium, "Through the Looking Glass: Reflections of the Past and Visions of the Future."

In recognizing the human limitations that affect people's ability to forecast the future, I acknowledge that the mirror into which we search for a glimpse of the future is opaque. For the vision reflected in the mirror of the future to become clear, we must listen, observe, evaluate, study, learn, and take action. Action that will influence the future requires taking risks. The symposium and the study described are among many steps needed to influence and direct a future of improved services for individuals who are blind or visually impaired.

The "force field" approach used by the study identified the items that were perceived as the most important and most likely events by most respondents. Through my work at the American Foundation for the Blind (AFB), I am also interested in the impact of some of the event statements that were not deemed critical by other respondents in the study. Therefore, in this chapter I discuss some of the event statements not addressed in the last phase of the study in an effort to stimulate further contemplation and action by readers.

INCREASED KNOWLEDGE OF ASSESSMENT STRATEGIES, NEUROLOGICAL FUNCTIONING, AND LEARNING STYLES AND THE DEVELOPMENT OF AIDS

Four events, when conceived as occurring concurrently, will be mutually supportive and will ultimately have a significant effect upon the ability of individuals with low vision to maximize their use of visual information. These events were presented in Event Statement 1 ("An increased understanding of brain and neurological functioning as it relates to sight and seeing has resulted in improved methods of teaching the visually impaired"), Event Statement 17 ("The knowledge of how children with low vision learn has been greatly expanded; therefore, teachers of the visually handicapped devote more service delivery time to teaching the use of available vision"), Event Statement 25 ("Sophisticated assessments allow the effect of vision to be distinguished from other disabilities present in the multihandicapped child"), and Event Statement 6 ("Reductions in cost and size of low vision aids, along with added versatility, have permitted these aids to be 'programmed' [computerized] to meet individualized needs, pathologies, and/or tasks").

It is critical that research on neurology; learning styles and strategies of low vision learners, including those with multiple disabilities; and the development of low vision aids be expanded. The present barriers to information sharing among various types of service providers and between those in the for-profit sector and those in the educational and other areas of the nonprofit sector must be eradicated. Researchers in optics, developers of low vision aids, individuals with low vision, neurologists, teachers, ophthalmologists and optometrists, occupational therapists, psychologists, orientation and mobility specialists, and other service providers need to establish closer cooperation not only to stimulate the development of optical aids, but to improve the dissemination, availability, application, and quality of instruction in use of aids.

Low vision aids need to be distributed with instructional and user materials in print, audio, and video formats. These materials should be developed cooperatively with individuals with low vision, including children and adults, who will benefit from the use of the aids, as well as with parents and other family members, teachers of children and adults, orientation and mobility (O&M) specialists, and other professionals who will provide instruction and support the use of the aids. Furthermore, the results of research on aids, learning styles, and instructional strategies must be disseminated through publications and presentations in pre- and in-service training programs.

It is common practice for students and clients with low vision to receive significantly less specialized instruction from teachers who are certified in the education and rehabilitation of blind and visually impaired children and adults than do those who are blind. Often, the decision about how many hours per week a student or client will receive special education and rehabilitation services is made solely on the basis of the extent of the physiological disability. Therefore, research is clearly needed to determine whether this practice is widespread and its effects are beneficial or injurious. It is believed by some that if teachers and rehabilitation specialists were more knowledgeable, skilled, and confident in their abilities to assess visual limitations and capabilities accurately and to teach students and clients how to maximize their visual ability, both while using and not using optical aids, they would recognize the need to devote more time to teaching individuals with low vision.

It has been estimated that 23 million Americans are functionally illiterate and that as much as 65 percent of the work force is "intermediately" illiterate, that is, can read materials only at the fifth- to ninth-grade levels. Yet, most materials in the workplace are written at the 12th-grade level (Charlier, 1990). By 2000, below-average skills will be acceptable for only 27 percent of the jobs in this country, compared with 40 percent of the jobs in the mid-1980s, and 41 percent of the new jobs will require average or better levels of skills (Swasy & Hymowitz, 1990). Therefore, it is not surprising that improving the level of literacy in this country is an urgent task and will continue to be so as the required reading level continues to increase during coming decades of the information age.

Clearly, the literacy movement has had, and will continue to have, lasting and significant benefits for society. The National Federation of the Blind is requesting that state legislatures pass "braille bills," which would require the availability of braille instruction to every visually handicapped child if his or her parents want it. It is, however, imperative that each visually impaired individual's needs (both short- and long-term), capabilities, and limitations be carefully assessed. Braille is an appropriate reading medium for some visually impaired persons, but not for others. As Susan Spungin (quoted in De Witt, 1991, p. 1) said: "If you can read white dots on white paper with your eyes, then it is probably not appropriate to learn braille."

Thus, it is important that we give up the notion of teaching only one or the other reading mode. For some, braille is the most efficient and effective primary reading and writing mode, whereas audiotapes will be the secondary mode. For others, regular-size print in conjunction with optical aids, audiotapes, and braille may be the most effective and efficient combination of communication modes. People are capable not only of learning alternate reading modes concurrently, but of determining which reading mode or modes may be the best for their various reading needs. In addition, it is important to realize that the primary reading medium and supplementary secondary learning media may change as students' or clients' visual ability and visual tasks change (Mangold & Mangold, 1989). To make these determinations, both children and adults must be comfortable with the idea that they can learn and use various modes at different times and for different purposes.

Today, you can go to a hair salon or a plastic surgeon's office and see on a computer screen what you would look like with different hair styles, noses, mouths, chins, and so on. In the future, technology will provide us with accurate assessments and simulations of exactly what each individual with low vision sees on the basis of his or her specific visual etiology and impairment and the effects of various low vision aids in combination with those specific and unique visual capabilities and limitations. Our assessments, prescriptive processes, and low vision aids will be greatly improved, and we will be less dependent on how well we interpret what students or clients describe as their visual capabilities or cannot communicate because of their multiple impairments.

However, the psychosocial aspects of the application of technological advancements will not be as instantly apparent or remedied. As Naisbitt (1984) noted, the more technology is introduced into our lives, the more we will need contact and support from other people. The human factors that motivate our students and clients to cope, to learn, and to apply knowledge and skills will remain critical variables that service providers must consider and deal with sensitively. The need for research and for the development of strategies and the effective application of counseling theory and support systems will continue. It will be through mutual and collaborative efforts among individuals with low vision and their families, researchers, eye care specialists, neurologists, educators, and other service providers that educational theories, strategies, and devices for the utilization of vision and the assessment and enhancement of low vision will become more sophisticated and will be more widely applied in the future.

THE INCREASED PREVALENCE OF LOW VISION AMONG ELDERLY PERSONS

Research has supported the first part of Event Statement 10, that the "increased prevalence of low vision among the aging population has resulted in greater acceptance of individuals with visual impairment." During the 1980s, the number of Americans aged 65 and over increased by 24 percent, almost 2.5 times the growth in the general population (Orr, 1992). Every day, there are 1,600 additional older adults in this country (Denton, 1990). By 2000, persons over age 65 will represent 13 percent of the total population (American Association of Retired Persons, 1990). "Today's 65 plus population of 31.5 million is projected to reach 34.9 million in 2000, 39.4 million in 2010, 52.1 million in 2020, 65.6 million in 2030, and a peak of 68.5 million in 2050" (National Council on the Aging, 1991, p.4).

In 1979, it was projected that from 1977 to 2000, the number of elderly persons with severe visual impairments would increase from 990,000 to 1,760,000 (Kirchner, 1985). However, national data collected in the late 1980s demonstrated that the prevalence of visual impairment among elderly people is "at least twice as great as the number suggested" (Nelson, 1987, p. 334). The fastest-growing segment of the elderly population is persons aged 85 and older (Crews, 1991). The National Council on the Aging (1991) forecasts that there will be 15.3 million persons aged 85 and over in 2050, up from 3.5 million in 1991. Furthermore, the "number of severely visually impaired older persons will increase from 2 million in 1980, to about 3.2 million in 2000, and to 4.6 million in 2020" (Crews, 1991, p. 52) and persons over age 85 will be the largest group of those with severe visual impairments—1.6 million by 2010, or about 1 in 4 of that age group (up from 560,000 in 1980). Therefore, the research is clear with respect to the rapid growth of the aging population, as well as of severely visually impaired persons among that population.

Where the event statement falls short is in the assumption that the increased number of visually impaired elderly people will change the public's attitudes toward those with visual impairments. If one looks at the public's attitudes toward other segments of the population that are growing significantly, such as persons who are homeless, mentally ill, poor, or have AIDS, as well as members of minority groups, it is clear that increased prevalence does not bring about changes in attitudes or acceptance.

To date, there is no indication that the growing prevalence of elderly persons has resulted in greater acceptance of older persons or older persons who are visually impaired or any other group of elderly persons. Vision loss among the elderly is associated with the aging process, and it is the aging process itself that continues to be perceived negatively by American society.

The present and anticipated increased rates of prevalence of older persons with Alzheimer's disease and older persons with vision loss are nearly parallel, yet the public remains unaware of and indifferent to the effects of vision loss and the consequent needs of and appropriate rehabilitation services for elderly persons who are visually impaired. In contrast, since the 1980s, there has been a massive and consistent public education and public policy campaign regarding Alzheimer's disease. Today, most Americans know that Alzheimer's disease is a form of dementia; that it is debilitating and progressive; and that there is a great need for research, funding, treatment, and family and societal support. Knowledge frequently leads to greater understanding, and since the public now knows significantly more about Alzheimer's disease than it did 10 years ago, it is more likely to support changes in public policy and increased funding for the research on and treatment of the disease than it did then. Similarly strong public education or public policy campaigns to alert the public to the needs of elderly persons with vision loss are essential for Event Statement 10 to become a reality.

Service providers in the field of blindness need to replicate programs for the elderly that have demonstrated success, as has been done with programs for people with Alzheimer's disease. Nationally recognized programs that highlight the capabilities of elderly persons must include elderly persons who are blind or visually impaired. For example, elderly blind and visually impaired individuals who have the desire and potential to serve as foster grandparents should be encouraged to do so. Not only could they serve as mentors for children with visual impairments, reinforcing their braille-reading skills, serving as role models, and giving them information about various careers, but they could be mentors or foster grandparents to nondisabled children as well. Furthermore, elderly blind and visually impaired people should be included as volunteers and salaried workers in programs where they can utilize their wealth of experience while contributing to the growth of others and enjoying the benefits of such programs. It is through positive contact with others who are different from us that we can change our unwarranted biases. Therefore, this society must make a concerted effort not only to improve services and opportunities for elderly persons, but to change negative attitudes toward persons who are elderly and blind or visually impaired.

EQUAL AND IMMEDIATE ACCESS TO INFORMATION

Few, if any, would dispute that in comparison with sighted individuals, those who are blind or have low vision never have had, nor do they presently have, equal and immediate access to information. Whether we consider "traditional" or "technological" sources of information, such as books, newspapers, or electronic mail systems, there is no doubt that information systems have been developed for access by sighted individuals and that these systems were then modified and/or devices were developed to provide access to those with visual impairments. Such methods have included the braille codes, enlarged print, optical aids, speech output, Talking Books, talking newspapers, speech synthesizers, and audiodescription. However, there is usually a significant time lag between the availability of information and information delivery systems and the development of modifications or systems for visually impaired persons. Instead of equal access after the fact, it would be preferable for access to be ensured from the start.

With regard to Event Statement 5, that "automatic bank teller machines and other graphic displays have been converted to large print and/or speech output for greater access to the visually impaired," the Americans with Disabilities Act (ADA) referred to automated teller machines (ATMs) and made four federal departments or agencies responsible for implementing the act. One such agency is the Architectural and Transportation Barriers Compliance Board (ATBCB), which issued proposed rules to guide the Department of Justice and the Department of Transportation concerning accessible design standards for buildings and facilities, transportation vehicles, and transportation facilities, as well as performance specifications to ensure the accessibility of public phones, ATMs, point-of-sale machines, and computer displays (Marshall, 1991). One of the proposed rules states that it would be a violation of Title III to build a new bank with ATMs that are not readily accessible to and usable by persons with disabilities ("Proposed Rules," 1991).

In response to the proposed rules and the proposed standards of the American National Standard Institute, AFB made the following recommendations (Ellis, 1991):

1. Assistive technology can create an interactive system whereby a user is aware of the specific responses of the ATMs while maintaining his or her privacy. A handset, with either live or recorded instructions, coupled with an appropriately marked key pad, could serve this purpose for most individuals who are blind or visually impaired, and braille instructions would be essential, particularly for those who are deaf-blind.

2. If instructions in the use of an ATM cannot be provided verbally through a permanently mounted handset, ATMs could be equipped with a jack and speech-synthesis technology to enable a customer to use a personal listening device (perhaps in the form of a Walkman-style headset) that could be plugged in and used as needed.

Handsets are already present on many existing ATMs. Furthermore, at least one ATM manufacturer is investigating the use of synthetic speech output for its ATM machines. In addition, braille instruction plaques for various models of ATM machines and braille ATM usage brochures have been designed and are available in limited quantities to financial institutions through the efforts of a volunteer braille project in Texas.

3. Glare problems at outdoor ATMs could be reduced by the addition of a hood or visor over the screen. Visually impaired users would also be aided by a high-contrast color display that could be switched to large characters on demand. The customer's ATM card could also be encoded in a manner that could toggle the machine into its accessible mode. As an adjunct to accessible ATM service, a record of account activity could be provided to the customer in either braille or large print. A few financial institutions around the country, notably the Chemical Bank of New York, currently provide braille or large-print statements to their blind or visually impaired customers (Marshall & Joffee, 1991).

In the future, technology will address many other areas related to access to public transportation, such as access to maps, timetables, route information, and self-ticketing at point of sale used by many mass transit systems. The ADA will motivate industry to develop accessible technology. In addition to legislation, what is needed is a heightened awareness, concern, and commitment by information producers with respect to the needs of blind and visually impaired persons. We need to strive toward a day when information systems are developed for use by all individuals with equal access *at the time of development*.

INTERAGENCY COORDINATION OF INFORMATION AND SERVICES

Event Statement 14, "Improved computer data base management has resulted in interagency (i.e., APH [American Printing House for the Blind], Library of Congress, RFB [Recording for the Blind], etc.) coordination and more effective tracking and programming for visually impaired children" was considered highly desirable, likely to occur, and of high impact. The key word in this statement is *interagency*.

As Spungin (1990, p. 11) stated:

> "The lack of a centralized source of information for the easy
> location of books in special formats for blind and visually
> handicapped persons in this day and age is incomprehensible.
> Despite the proliferation of database systems, the reading needs of
> blind and visually handicapped people rely, for the most part, on
> an informal system of literature search that is usually dependent on
> the help of sighted persons."

Major attempts are being made to ensure the development of comprehensive and compatible data-base systems. In 1984 the AFB Networking Taskforce was developed to investigate the extent of the duplication of efforts to produce materials in alternate formats and to develop recommendations to facilitate the establishment of either a comprehensive central listing system or compatible systems. As a result, the Coalition for Information Access for Print Handicapped Readers (CIAPHR) was established in 1988. It is CIAPHR's mission to address the persistent problems related to the location of and access to reading materials for blind and visually impaired persons. CIAPHR is committed to exploring the feasibility and means of developing a comprehensive listing system for all materials produced in braille, large print, and recorded form in North America and is developing guidelines and liaisons with producers, disseminators, and holders of such materials.

The National Library Service (NLS) for the Blind and Physically Handicapped of the Library of Congress recognizes "that there should be a single catalog that would include the non-NLS-produced books held at regional libraries and elsewhere in the world. Access to materials . . . would be greatly increased if the holdings of many institutions could be checked by searching one catalog" (NLS, 1990, p. 2). Presently, NLS is accepting title entries from Recording for the Blind (RFB), as well as from holdings in Canada, Australia, and Japan. RFB is accepting title entries from other producers of materials in alternate formats, and the American Printing House for the Blind (APH) is expanding its data-base capability to demonstrate its commitment to list titles from other agencies. Therefore, there is considerable reason to believe that the development and application of a standardized data-entry system will significantly improve access to information and provide a means by which individuals who are blind and visually impaired will be able to gain direct access to one data base to determine the availability, location, and format of any book.

The development and utilization of a standardized data-entry system must be coupled with additional strategies to make the event statement fully achievable, particularly the phrase that such efforts would lead to "more effective tracking and programming for visually impaired children." Systems and cooperative agreements must be established, not only among national organizations that collect information about children who are blind or visually impaired, but also with consumer organizations, parent-support groups, state and local education agencies, and resource centers for instructional materials. If the field is ever to have dependable and irrefutable data on the prevalence of various forms of visual impairment and the characteristics of the population, we will need to share information that can be combined and be free of duplication. Such data are critical to forecasting because they provide the information for analysis that will lead to the identification of trends and needs that will serve as the blueprints for the development of effective programs.

Virginia passed legislation in 1990 that could be a model for the nation. This legislation included a request to study the need to require schools to offer braille instruction in their special education programs and, in cooperation with the Department for the Visually Handicapped of Virginia, to evaluate the role of braille instruction as a viable method of promoting literacy among all blind and visually impaired students in the commonwealth. The Virginia Board of Education was charged with determining the number of blind students who could benefit from braille instruction but who were not receiving it, the appropriateness of requiring that braille instruction should be offered to such students according to their individualized education programs, and the concurrent increases in cost associated with such instruction. The board was further charged with determining the need to promulgate regulations requiring that braille instruction be offered in the special education programs and the need for instructional and administrative organization, instructional and support personnel, preservice and in-service training, and resources to support the implementation of any recommendations regarding the provision of instruction in reading braille (Virginia Senate, 1990). Such legislation supports categorical identification and recognizes the unique needs of visually impaired children.

In June 1991, landmark legislation was signed in Texas, stating that

> "the Central Education Agency shall require a publisher of a
> textbook adopted by the State Board of Education to furnish the
> agency with computer diskettes for literary subjects in the
> American Standard Code for Information Interchange (ASCII)
> from which braille versions of the textbook can be produced. The
> publisher will furnish the agency with computer diskettes in ASCII
> for non-literary subjects, e.g., natural sciences, computer science,
> mathematics and music, when Braille specialty code translation
> software is available" (Texas House Bill, 1991, p. 2).

This legislation also included a mandate to establish a commission to expedite its implementation. Activities of the commission are to include the development of processes and software for converting formatted textbook files to ASCII required for braille translation software and study the feasibility of implementing a process by which textbook publishers can transmit data files via modems directly to the computers of organizations that produce masters of braille textbooks. This legislation and the work of the commission will result in a significantly reduced time lapse in transforming print materials into braille for blind students in one state. The precedent set by Texas must be replicated in other states until such action is required and practiced throughout the nation. Work has since progressed with textbook publishers and major producers of books in braille and audiotape, such as APH and RFB.

THIRD-PARTY PAYMENTS FOR SERVICES

Third-party reimbursements for educational and rehabilitation services is a new, evolving, and highly complex area. The respondents to the survey were secure in their belief that Event Statement 21, that "low vision and vision rehabilitation specialist services are covered by insurance and health care providers as part of standard medical practice," would occur. But it will not happen without major and concerted efforts in multiple areas. Tied to third-party payments is the need for licensing and certification programs, as well as for the development of policies at the national level for all citizens, within state rehabilitation systems and state education systems and local school districts. New directions in national health care reform

110

during and following the Clinton administration will also be critical factors in the fulfillment of this event statement.

Stotland stated that "families in the year 2014 . . . should be receiving a far more positive view" of what their visually impaired child's life can be (see Chapter 3). But we continue to hear horror stories from parents of physicians who recommend institutionalization of babies who are blind or the withholding of intrusive medical procedures to save these babies' lives (Huebner & Ferrell, 1985). We cannot ignore the needs of infants and toddlers who are blind or visually impaired, including those with multiple disabilities. Consider the Head Start program, which was initially authorized under the Economic Opportunity Act of 1964 (Braddock, 1987). Granted, it took many years before the Head Start program was able to prove the positive impact of early intervention on child development. Yet, did the field of special education or the field of blindness take notice and act to develop similar interventions for this age group of children with disabilities? It was not until the Economic Opportunity Act Amendments of 1972, P.L. 92-424, that policies and procedures were established to ensure that not less than 10 percent of those enrolled in the Head Start Program would be children with disabilities. Now this policy is under threat and requires advocacy to retain it.

In 1989, the International Center for the Disabled reported that "the majority of both principals and teachers have not had adequate training in special education, and many are not very confident in making decisions concerning handicapped children" (p. 5). Few university personnel preparation programs specializing in blindness have been modified to include curricula and requirements in the area of early childhood or multiple disabilities. Yet, the need existed long before the first personnel preparation programs were begun and long before the passage of P.L. 94-142 in 1975 or P.L. 99-457 in 1986. Has the field of blindness initiated a national and inclusive program to address the needs of infants and toddlers who are blind or visually impaired, including those with multiple disabilities?

Barraga stated in her presentation that the critical factors that influenced past changes in philosophy and practice "center around general attitudes in the field, terminology, organizations and their journals, strategic events, teacher education, and research and literature" (see Chapter 1). Have we been slow to recognize emerging trends and been resistant to modifying practices?

Is the field so steeped in tradition that we find greater comfort in continuing with things as they are, rather than in taking risks to achieve change? We cannot hope to influence the future of services for individuals who are blind or visually impaired without considering present and future social, educational, industrial, medical, economic, and political trends, as well as trends that may be unique to the field of blindness.

Some social factors that will affect future generations of individuals who are blind or visually impaired, their families, and service providers were identified in Chapters 3 and 5. These factors should not be ignored, because they are related to the decisions that must be made and the actions that must be taken if we are to effect change and thereby influence the future direction of the field. Additional societal event statements to be considered include the following:

- More than 50 percent of the babies born today are born to teenage mothers (Whitted, 1987).

- Teenage pregnancies are on the rise (United Way of America, 1987).

- The number of single-parent families will increase (Wilson, 1987).

- High poverty rates in female-headed families will continue (United Way of America, 1987; Wilson, 1987).

- The proportion of minority students is increasing while the proportion of minority teachers is decreasing (Carnegie Forum, 1986).

- The shortage of university professors and public school teachers is increasing, accompanied by a greater interest in improving the quality of personnel (Head, 1989; McLaughlin, Smith-Davis, & Burke, 1986; Silberman, Corn, & Sowell, 1989; United Way of America, 1987).

- A greater proportional growth in the minority population (United Way of America, 1987; Whitted, 1987) will require social service personnel to apply knowledge and strategies that are sensitive to ethnic, cultural, and linguistic differences (Huebner, 1989).

- Issues related to drug abuse will continue to escalate (William T. Grant Foundation, 1988) and will effect educational, health, and rehabilitation policies.

- The AIDS epidemic will have a substantial impact on education, rehabilitation, human rights, and policy development (Huebner, 1989).

- The decentralization of the government from the federal to the state and local levels will continue (Toffler, 1980; United Way of America, 1987; Wilson, 1987).

- Health care reform will have an impact on services and the way they are delivered.

Barraga opened the symposium by reflecting on memories—what they are, what they mean to us, and how they come about. The challenge before us is to expand our perspectives, take risks, and act. We are obliged to observe, study, and learn from other fields, and not just those related to disabilities or social services. If Dr. Richard Hoover had limited his interest to ophthalmology, would there be a long cane or the profession of O&M? If John Linville and Jim Bliss had not been interested in both the technology emerging from NASA and the needs of individuals who are blind, would we have the Optacon or other technological devices developed at TeleSensory Corporation?

We are also challenged to develop and provide educational and rehabilitation services that take into account the entire individual—not just a person's academic, social and emotional, skills, health, or economic needs, but all the facets of each individual. The field of education and rehabilitation for individuals who are blind or visually impaired has a rich history of progressive practice, but much remains to be done. Every event statement identified in the papers presented at the symposium and those investigated during the study require both individual and collaborative efforts to be realized. Every event statement requires both individual professional growth and change, as well as change in the system.

REFERENCES

American Association of Retired Persons. (1990). *A profile of older Americans.* Washington, DC: Author.

American Foundation for the Blind. (1991 Internal Document). *Mission statement.* New York, N.Y.: Author.

Braddock, D. (1987). *Federal policy toward mental retardation and developmental disabilities.* Baltimore, MD: Paul H. Brookes.

Carnegie Forum on Education and the Economy. (1986, May). *A nation prepared: Teachers for the 21st century. The Report of the Task Force on Teaching as a Profession.* New York: Author.

Cetron, M., & O'Toole, T. (1982). *Encounters with the future: A forecast of life into the 21st century.* New York: McGraw-Hill.

Charlier, M. (1990, February 9). Back to basics: Businesses try to teach their workers the three R's since schools have failed to do so. *Wall Street Journal,* pp. R14–R15.

Crews, J.E. (1991). Strategic planning and independent living for elders who are blind. *Journal of Visual Impairment & Blindness, 85,* 52–57.

Denton, D. R. (1990). *Caring for an aging society: Issues and strategies for gerontology education.* (Available from Southern Regional Education Board, 592 10th Street, NW, Atlanta, GA 30318-5790.)

De Witt, K. (1991, May 12). How best to teach the blind: A growing battle over braille. *New York Times,* pp. 1, 4.

Ellis, F. J. (1991). The Politics of access for blind and visually impaired persons. *AFB News, 26*(1), 5.

Head, D. N. (1989). The future of low incidence training programs: A national problem. *RE:view, 21,* 145–152.

Huebner, K. M. (1989). Shaping educational intervention for blind and visually impaired learners in response to social change. *RE:view, 21,* 137–144.

Huebner, K. M. & Ferrell, K. A. (1985). Ethical practice in providing services to blind and visually impaired students. In *Ethical issues in the field of blindness* (pp. 9-20). New York: American Foundation for the Blind.

114

International Center for the Disabled. (1989). *The ICD Survey III: A report card on special education*. New York: Louis Harris & Associates.

Kirchner, C. (1985). *Data on blindness and visual impairment in the U.S.: A resource manual on social demographic characteristics, education, employment and income, and service delivery*. New York: American Foundation for the Blind.

Mangold, S., & Mangold, P. (1989). Selecting the most appropriate primary learning medium for students with functional vision. *Journal of Visual Impairment & Blindness, 83,* 294-296.

Marshall, S. (1991). AFB offers perspective concerning proposed ADA regulations. *Network Report, 2*(2), 1-4.

Marshall, S., & Joffee, E. (1991). Unpublished comments of the American Foundation for the Blind, submitted to the Architectural and Transportation Barriers Compliance Board, March 25, 1991, in response to Notice of Proposed Rule Making, Americans with Disabilities Act Accessibility Guidelines for Buildings and Facilities as published in the Federal Register, January 22, 1991, 56 FR 2296, Docket No. 90-2; 36 CFR 1191.

McLaughlin, M. J., Smith-Davis, J., & Burke, P. J. (1986). *Personnel to educate the handicapped in America: A status report*. College Park, MD: University of Maryland, College of Special Education, Institute for the Study of Exceptional Children and Youth.

Naisbitt, J. (1984). *Megatrends*. New York: Warner Books.

National Council on the Aging. (1991). The aging revolution. *In Perspective on Aging: NCOA annual report* (pp. 4-5). Washington, DC: Author.

National Library Service for the Blind and Physically Handicapped of the Library of Congress. (1990). *"Cataloging for access" in projects and experiments*. Washington, DC: Author.

Nelson, K. A. (1987). Visual impairment among elderly Americans: Statistics in transition. *Journal of Visual Impairment & Blindness, 81,* 331-334.

Orr, A. (1992). Aging and blindness: Toward a systems approach to service delivery. In A. L. Orr (Ed.), *Vision and aging: Crossroads for service delivery* (pp. 3-31). New York: American Foundation for the Blind.

Proposed rules. (1991, January 22). *Federal Register, 58*(14), 2314.

Silberman, R. K., Corn, A. L., & Sowell, V. M. (1989). A Profile of teacher educators and the future of their personnel preparation programs for serving visually handicapped children and youth. *Journal of Visual Impairment & Blindness, 83,* 150-155.

Spungin, S. J. (1990). *Braille literacy: Issues for blind persons, families, professionals, and producers of braille*. New York: American Foundation for the Blind.

Swasy, A., & Hymowitz, C. (1990, February 9). The workplace revolution. *Wall Street Journal.* pp. R6–R8.

Texas House Bill No. 2277, Section 3, 12.03, e. (1991, June 13).

Toffler, A. (1980). *The new wave.* New York: Bantam Books.

United Way of America. (1987). *What lies ahead: Looking toward the 90's.* (Available from Strategic Planning Division, 701 North Fairfax Street, Alexandria, VA 22314.)

Virginia Senate Joint Resolution No. 36 (1990). Commonwealth of Virginia. Resolution agreed by the Senate March 9, 1990 and by the House of Delegates, March 7, 1990.

Whitted, E. (1987). Keynote address presented at the Futures Conference, Council for Exceptional Children, Orlando, FL.

William T. Grant Foundation. (1988). *William T. Grant Foundation annual report 1987.* New York: Author.

Wilson, W. J. (1987). *The truly disadvantaged: The inner city, the underclass, and public policy.* Chicago: University of Chicago Press.

Chapter 12

CAN WE GET THERE FROM HERE?

Virginia E. Bishop, Ph.D.

University of Texas at Austin

The symposium entitled "Through the Looking Glass: Reflections of the Past and Visions of the Future" sought to identify issues of importance in planning for the future of individuals who are blind or visually impaired. The study took the issues and examined them further, using a forecasting approach called force-field analysis. The intent was to identify developments that would have the greatest impact on persons who are blind or visually impaired and on the forces that would enable them to occur if they were desirable or would prevent them from occurring if they were undesirable. People who had experience or knowledge in the field of visual impairment projected that the final five developments would be the most important and presented strategies for effecting the desired outcomes. However, action that will influence the future requires planning, a unified and organized effort, and a willingness to take risks. Nothing of value is ever attained without risk and effort. If we who are interested in the future of individuals who are blind or visually impaired can pool our thinking, efforts, and energies, we *can* have an impact on what the future will bring.

This final chapter examines the issues, strategies, and goals and presents a structured approach to influencing the future. If we are to effect change and/or improvement in services for individuals who are blind or visually impaired, we *must* take action. We are no less creative or energetic than our predecessors. A generation from now, may they say of us that we met the challenge and won.

EVALUATION OF STATEMENTS

A number of the original statements were evaluated by the study participants and discarded from future examination. The statements were discarded for one of two reasons. First, the respondents thought that some statements were highly unlikely; for example, orientation and mobility (O&M) instruction will *never* be standardized, since it is so highly individualized; low vision specialists are *already* separate from education as a profession; the invention of artificial vision systems for blind people is probably not within the 25-year projection period; teachers of the visually impaired will always be teachers, affiliated with an educational system, and not private practitioners; elderly visually impaired people are not likely to speak up loudly enough to become a powerful political force; and teachers of the visually impaired are not ever likely to be paid higher salaries. Second, the respondents thought that even if the events in some statements occurred, the impact would not be that great; for instance, even if the number of minority professionals were to increase, their greater number probably would not affect the quality or quantity of services provided; a national program of evaluation, accreditation, or accountability would probably not improve services that much; even if computers were able to simulate visual experience by interpreting brain waves, functional vision evaluations would probably continue to provide more comprehensive data for planning; and even if a national health care plan was instituted, people with visual problems would probably still be underreferred and underserved. One issue—the relationship between disability labels and individual assessments—the opinions of the respondents were so polarized that this issue will be discussed later. Since this study polled a large number of professionals, no attempt will be made to contradict their collective opinion on the issues they deemed to be unlikely or ineffective.

The remaining 12 issues were examined in more depth in the second phase of the study. Of the 12, 9 were considered desirable by a large majority of the participants, two were viewed as undesirable by the same majority, and one had a one-third–two-thirds split in favor of undesirability. When examining the force fields, however, the investigator found that for five of the desirable issues, strong forces were already in place that would ensure their occurrence; that is, alternatives to graphic displays will become commonplace; improved technology will decrease the size and cost of low vision devices; because there will be a greater number of elderly people with visual impairments, their increased visibility will make their disabilities more acceptable; interagency data sharing will result from improved computerized data-based management; and there is every likelihood that there will be more information on how children with low vision learn.

Of the remaining four desirable events (which will be discussed later), two had minimal but adequate forces to produce the desired result; thus, health care insurance will *probably* be expanded to cover low vision and vision rehabilitation services, and assessments of children with multiple handicaps will *probably* be able to separate out the effects of a visual impairment from the effects of the other disabilities. The other two desirable events—increased knowledge of brain function and specialized certification of selected early childhood teachers—had weak forces that place them at risk of occurrence. Both the undesirable events had weak facilitating forces; that is, the restraining forces were not strong enough to prevent the undesirable outcomes. The issue that produced a split opinion also had a split weighting of forces, with an advantage to the facilitating forces; more people saw it as undesirable, but more people thought that the forces would cause it to occur anyway. All the last three event statements will be discussed as part of this final summary section.

RECOMMENDATIONS FOR ACTION

Since the purpose of this final section is to translate the study data into a plan for action, each of the seven event statements mentioned previously will be discussed with that goal in mind. Strategies proposed by the study participants will be combined into recommended actions and summarized as proposals. The reader is challenged to implement the suggested plans.

Statement 1

An increased understanding of brain and neurological functioning, as it relates to sight and seeing, has resulted in improved methods of teaching the visually impaired.

It has been said that the brain may be one of the future's final frontiers. The rapid expansion of knowledge about how the brain works may be one of science's most important contributions to education and rehabilitation. The brain's role in vision and in visual functioning is central to the learning process, and every discovery about the brain can yield new insights into the understanding of visual functioning. However, if this knowledge is not translated into practice, particularly in the field of learning theory, the possibilities may be confined to treatments. Therefore, it is urgent that educators learn what is new in neurology and neuroanatomy by keeping abreast of the latest research. It is also important for educators and scientists (including neurologists, ophthalmologists, and psychologists) to respect each other's disciplines and to communicate openly with each other. Only then will both science and education profit from any new discoveries.

Recommendations

1. Plan reciprocal in-service courses for educators and scientists, with each discipline contributing information on a specific topic. The educator may contribute observations of how vision affects learning, whereas the scientist may describe how different parts of the brain affect vision or visual behaviors. These in-service courses should be held annually, perhaps in connection with relevant conferences.

2. Plan reciprocal field trips. Teachers may visit hospitals or neurologists' or ophthalmologists' offices, whereas physicians or interns could spend a day in a special education classroom.

3. Include guest lectures by teachers in medical internships and guest lectures by physicians and researchers in teacher preparation courses.

4. Interchange reports; for example, functional vision evaluations should be sent to ophthalmologists and neurological reports should be shared with teachers. Observe confidentiality regulations strictly.

5. Include an ophthalmologist and/or a neurologist on an educational team, utilizing interdisciplinary approaches to evaluations. Allow the teacher of the visually impaired to be present during the child's visual or neurological examination.

6. Try out interdisciplinary internships, such as a teacher with an ophthalmologist and a neurologist with a teacher.

7. Encourage physicians to visit their patients in school settings.

8. Monitor medical journals, watching for research reports that have implications for visual functioning.

9. Begin research report columns in professional vision journals, with findings presented in user-friendly terms.

10. Plan and implement joint research projects between scientists and educators, with findings that have implications for education included in the final report.

11. Require that graduate students in certification programs for teachers of the visually impaired read and report on current research in science and/or medicine.

12. Create a national clearinghouse for research. The primary function of the clearinghouse should be the dissemination of research findings that may have an impact on the field of vision, particularly in the area of brain function.

Statement 2

Child care and early intervention programs for visually impaired children are required to have specially certified teachers.

Early childhood legislation now requires all preschool children with disabilities to be located and served, according to their and their families' needs. Since very young children may be difficult to assess, especially in areas of sensory impairments, the expertise of the teacher of the visually impaired is essential. In special education programs where such a teacher may be employed, this expertise may be available, but in rural or poor school districts, it may not. Because the generic early childhood–early intervention (EC-EI) teacher usually does not have specific training in the impact of a visual impairment on early development and may not be able to differentiate between maturational delay and the effects of a visual impairment, intervention time could be lost, and such time is rarely regained. There is a need for both early childhood teachers and teachers of the visually impaired to have cross-disciplinary training. Although it would be desirable to have a separate certification for a teacher trained in both areas, that goal may be unrealistic in light of the critical shortage of teachers of the visually impaired. Therefore, the most practical solution would seem to be cross-disciplinary training.

Recommendations

1. Include at least one course at the preservice level that is cross-disciplinary and require both EC-EI teachers and teachers of the visually impaired to take the course.

2. Include at least one lecture on vision and early development in courses for nurses, neonatologists, and rehabilitation counselors.

3. Plan cross-disciplinary in-service courses for both EC-EI teachers and teachers of the visually impaired. These should be at least one-day presentations on normal childhood development and intervention methods (for teachers of the visually impaired) and on the impact of a visual impairment on early development (for EC-EI teachers).

4. Produce and disseminate public awareness documents and/or announcements that emphasize the importance of early intervention for infants and young children with visual impairments. Target school administrators, directors of special education, and the general public for exposure to this information.

5. Accumulate research data on how a visual impairment affects early development. Disseminate this information to both EC-EI teachers and teachers of the visually impaired.

6. Include a teacher of the visually impaired on the consulting staffs of neonatal units and pediatric ophthalmologists' offices.

7. Conduct cross-exceptionality workshops at local, state, and national conferences, to make both EC-EI teachers and teachers of the visually impaired aware of current trends, cooperative service models, and interdisciplinary approaches to working with families.

8. Include at least one lecture in teacher preparation courses for teachers of the visually impaired on working with families (especially at the preschool level, where family needs are incorporated into the educational plan). Require accompanying fieldwork, preferably in cooperation with a certified EC-EI teacher.

9. Encourage teachers of the visually impaired to minor in EC-EI. Plan reciprocal programs between universities, to allow the exchange of instructors.

10. Utilize residential schools in the summer for cross-disciplinary experience and training in working with preschool children who are visually impaired. Inviting parents to attend for at least one day could provide experience in working with families.

11. Enlist the help of parents (through NAPVI) in asking for appropriate services. When a child is visually impaired, he or she requires the early intervention expertise of a teacher of the visually impaired as soon as the visual impairment has been noticed or identified.

12. Prepare informational pamphlets for distribution in baby clinics, hospitals, pediatricians' offices, and offices of pediatric ophthalmologists. These documents should describe the impact of a visual impairment on early development and the need for special intervention services from a certified teacher of the visually impaired.

13. Advocate for disability-specific services at all educational levels, but especially at the preschool level. These preschool years are a critical time for children with visual impairments to learn.

14. Encourage administrators to maintain disability-specific head-count records (even though such head counts are not required by law). If administrators are made aware of the number of visually impaired preschool children, they are more likely to hire teachers who are trained to serve these children and can rationalize the teachers' employment.

15. Consider a mobile classroom (a specially equipped motor home or van) to serve young visually impaired children and their families in a broader geographic area.

16. Generate research data to support the claim that a generic EC-EI service is inadequate for infants and young children who are visually impaired. Disseminate the data to school administrators.

Statement 3

Due to increased litigation and bureaucratic constraints, teachers have less contact with families during the educational program planning process.

One of the major intents of P.L. 94-142 and its amendments was to include parents in the process of developing an Individualized Education Program (IEP). In some cases, it has worked well, but in others, parents are still "outsiders." Sometimes parents' disconnectedness is voluntary (they do not care or do not have time), but often it occurs because parents are intentionally kept poorly informed. These parents have had to resort to litigation to remain involved in their children's education. Other reasons why teachers have little contact with parents include excessive paperwork, large caseloads, and the lack of training in how to work with parents. When the IEP process becomes confrontational instead of inclusive and cooperative, the chief loser is the child. If educators are to have the greatest opportunity to facilitate learning in students who are visually impaired, there *must* be a positive, mutually respectful, and communicative relationship between teachers and parents in planning educational programs.

Recommendations

1. Include strategies for working cooperatively with parents in teacher preparation courses. Require some degree of supervised and applied fieldwork as a part of this training.

2. Plan and implement in-services programs or workshops for teachers of the visually impaired on how to work effectively with parents. Emphasize the contributions of parents as members of IEP teams. Include such topics as listening skills, conflict resolution, family dynamics, and communication skills in the programs.

3. Conduct informal retreats for parents, to help them meet other parents and to provide open forums for discussions of topics of interest to them. Provide child care services (perhaps staffed by student teachers) and family "fun" activities, to keep the interactions informal and nonthreatening.

4. Use a variety of parent-contact techniques (such as telephone calls, log books, daily notes or memos, regular conferences, and home visits) that are designed to meet the needs of individual families. Aim to spend as much time staying in touch with parents as in instructing the students.

5. Organize a group of parents who have children with visual impairments, and encourage them to meet regularly and to affiliate with NAPVI.

6. Prepare videotapes of children to share with parents. Allow the parents to view the tapes at home and encourage them to give feedback on the tapes. Do so at least three times each school year (at the beginning, in the middle, and at the end) to help document the children's progress.

7. Include parents on panels that are intended to help teachers know what parents want, feel, and need. (This can be done at the preservice or in-service level.)

8. Rewrite the local district's document that informs parents of their rights in terms that are understandable to the parents. Ask parents if they have any questions about what the document means and answer their questions honestly and simply.

9. Let parents know that their comments are welcome at the IEP planning meeting and that their concerns will be heard and included in the process. Establish a nonthreatening atmosphere in which to exchange ideas. Encourage parents to contribute evaluative information and work it into the final plan.

10. Plan and implement in-service programs for administrators regarding the importance of the parents and their concerns in the IEP process. When administrators view the process positively and openly, it is likely that others on the team (including the parents) will, too.

11. Include time for conferences and telephone calls with parents in teachers' schedules. Any formulas that compute caseloads based on services (rather than on head counts) should factor in time for contacts with parents.

12. Consider allowing compensatory time or flexitime for contacts with parents.

Statement 4

State schools and other institutions for the visually impaired serve only the most severely involved multiply handicapped children.

The role of the residential school for blind and visually impaired students has been debated for over 100 years. In the United States, it has gone from the only educational choice to one of a number of alternatives on a continuum of services. In addition, the kind of visually impaired children enrolled in residential schools has changed from "normal" to primarily visually impaired children with multiple handicaps. There seems to be little agreement, even among professionals, about the proper and most appropriate function of residential schools for blind and visually impaired students.

The respondents supported the *need* for residential schools (they should *not* be eliminated), but disagreed considerably on the *role* of such schools. This issue, more than any other, may reflect more about society, values, and the changing perception of special education than about education for visually impaired students. The deinstitutionalization philosophy touched residential schools, and students were returned to their homes and local schools. Only the more severely disabled children (for example, those who were deaf-blind or had multiple handicaps) were kept, largely because the public schools did not know what to do with them or how to educate them. As special education matured to include students with severe disabilities, even some of these children left the residential schools and returned to their home schools. As special education programs began to realize how specific the instructional methods could be for visually impaired students with multiple handicaps and how few specially trained teachers there were, many of these children were sent back to the residential schools for round-the-clock programming. Now, as "inclusion" threatens to place all disabled students in regular classrooms, residential schools must reexamine their roles, programs, and futures. This is an issue that requires the most unified, creative, innovative, determined, and philosophically sound resolution. Planning for the future is critical if residential schools are to survive.

Recommendations

1. Develop an exit-oriented philosophy (that is, that the residential school prepares a student for entering regular school or the "real world," whichever is most appropriate, depending on the child's age and acquired skills). This philosophy would encourage an expanded curriculum, more intensive instruction in skills, and more productive transitional planning. It would also encourage a sense of partnership between the residential school and the local school district as they worked jointly toward educating their students who are visually impaired.

2. Clarify the definition of least restrictive environment (LRE) in terms of most appropriate placement (MAP). Emphasize that the LRE-MAP may be other than mainstreaming for students who are visually impaired and may be the residential school.

3. Develop a means of determining the MAP. Devise a data-collection procedure to accumulate evidence that supports the recommended placement. If residential placement is determined to be the MAP, the documentation must prove that it is the best (if not the only) place the student can receive the recommended services.

4. Expand programs at residential schools to provide the following instructional services for students with visual impairments:

    a. Dual programs (for both "normal" students who are visually impaired and those who have additional disabilities).

b. Split placements (part-time mainstreaming at a local school and part-time day or residential placement, on a daily basis), with responsibilities to be shared between the local schools and the residential school.

c. Short-term (a year or less) intensive residential instruction in special (compensatory) skills.

d. Summer programs in specific skill areas (such as braille, computers, daily living skills, and O&M) for school-year mainstreamed students, with credit toward graduation offered for these courses.

e. A catch-up year between junior high school and high school or between high school graduation and college, to provide remedial instruction that will enable a smoother transition.

f. Model programs to demonstrate special techniques or for special populations.

5. Develop a plan to provide outreach services to local school districts across the state. Such services may include the following:

a. The provision of special training institutes for parents, regular educators, special educators, and teachers of the visually impaired.

b. Special training for school psychologists or diagnosticians in how to evaluate students who are visually impaired.

c. On-site special evaluations (of both students and programs).

d. On-site consultation for special problems.

e. The trial and/or loan of special equipment that is unique to students who are visually impaired.

6. Assume greater responsibility for teacher training and staff development by (a) cooperating with university teacher preparation programs to encourage observation and student teaching placements and (b) providing in-service programs and conducting seminars and/or conferences that expand or refine the skills of teachers of the visually impaired.

7. Act as a statewide resource for itinerant teachers of the visually impaired to answer specific questions and to disseminate research-based information.

8. Develop a series of curricula that can be used by both classroom teachers and itinerant teachers who are responsible for the instruction of students who are visually impaired. These curricula should not take the place of local school curricula, but should address the specific needs of students with visual impairments (such as special communication skills, daily living skills, social skills, O&M, and leisure-play skills).

9. Employ a staff of itinerant special teachers who can be sent to rural areas as needed—teachers whose home base is the residential school and who are professionally supervised by the residential school, but whose salary is shared by local schools according to the time the teachers spend in the district.

10. Devise a plan to set up regional centers (professional and/or instructional centers that are extensions of the residential school). Such centers would provide a variety of services similar to those provided by the residential school, but on a smaller scale.

11. Maintain a staff of specialists at the residential school with experience and training in a specialty area (such as braille instruction, technology, behavioral management, and assessment).

12. Act as a research center in the field of visual impairment. Collect data statewide on such topics as these:

    a. the changing etiologies of students with visual impairments

    b. evidence of success or failure in mainstreaming

    c. experimental methodologies with specific subgroups (for example, children who are deaf-blind or autistic or children with cortical visual impairments)

    d. trials of new technologies, under controlled conditions.

13. Disseminate research findings related to visual impairment (such as new information about the brain, new technology, and the medical management of ocular diseases and disorders).

Statement 5

Low vision and vision rehabilitation specialist services are covered by insurance and health care providers as part of standard medical practice.

The issue of third-party reimbursements for educational and rehabilitation services is an evolving and highly complex area of study. Although rehabilitation of individuals who are visually impaired has been publicly funded through state offices, it has not been fully covered by medical insurance. A few types of vision care (such as medical care and eyeglasses) are currently included in some health care plans, but the interpretations are not universal or standardized and may involve special premium payments or eligibility requirements. The situation in education is different, since few educational services for individuals with visual impairments are considered to be health related (and, thus, eligible for reimbursement under health care plans or insurance). Part of the problem involves the professional status of the providers. Physicians and opticians are considered to be professionals, whereas rehabilitation specialists and educators are not. The development of licensure and certification standards is necessary if reimbursement is to be viewed as appropriate. It may also be necessary to modify or change public policy at all levels—national, state, and local—within the rehabilitation and educational systems, to ensure the health care-insurance coverage of vision-related services.

Recommendations

1. Generate and agree on a definition of low vision. This definition is the essential first step toward the acceptance by policymakers and physicians of a distinct group of people who would be eligible for reimbursement.

2. Define those low vision services that would be eligible for reimbursement (for example, evaluation, the types and reasonable costs of low vision devices, and rehabilitation instruction in the use of these devices).

3. Establish strict licensing standards for professionals who provide low vision services (including optometrists or ophthalmologists who are low vision specialists and teachers who specialize in instructional methods for individuals with low vision).

4. Establish a system for monitoring the performance of specialists in low vision and a censure system when their performance is below standard or unethical. Include a means of controlling the billing of these professionals through a system of "reasonable and acceptable costs."

5. Create public awareness and educational programs that describe the effects of low vision on daily life, employment, and social interactions. Target audiences who are currently skeptical or uninformed about low vision (including the medical community, legislators, and the general public).

6. Demonstrate that the provision of low vision services and devices is cost effective. Show that such assistance increases the employability and productivity of individuals with low vision.

7. Unify the views of professionals through the creation of political alliances. Because of the low number of both consumers with low vision and professionals who serve them, it will be particularly important to present a unified and coordinated plan to pressure legislators, insurance providers, and other relevant groups to modify public policy to include low vision services and devices as reimbursable items in health care plans and health insurance. If this pressure can produce positive results, a broader plan of action may include a campaign to include low vision services in the Medicare list of reimbursable services.

Statement 6

Disability labels no longer exist relative to education; therefore, individualized assessment of specific disabilities is no longer required.

The generic special education model and the current movement toward "full inclusion" may not be in the best interests of students who are visually impaired. Although mainstreaming has always been, and will always be, one choice on the mandated continuum of service delivery models, it is not necessarily the only one, or even the preferred one, for students with visual impairments. Because a visual impairment can have a great impact on learning, the needs of these children can vary day to day and year to year. Special skills often cannot be taught in a regular classroom because the necessary instruction is so highly individualized and the regular education teacher (or the generic special education teacher) does not have the specialized training that is necessary to teach these skills. Special skills (such as braille, abacus, and special technology) and skills requiring specialized instructional techniques because of the visual impairment (including self-help, basic concepts, mobility, reasoning, and play) require baseline evaluations by a teacher trained in the area of visual impairment. Without this highly specialized knowledge, the assessment may be invalid and the results may be misinterpreted. If students have special needs related to a specific disability like visual impairment, they must be evaluated and instructed by a special teacher. To be eligible for these services, they must be determined to meet certain requirements. The result is a "disability label," which is unavoidable if appropriate services are to be provided.

Recommendations

1. Maintain a strong position advocating categorical services for students who are visually impaired. Such a stance requires a constant state of alertness, since the "full inclusion" movement is pressuring states and local school districts to disregard the mandates for a wide continuum of alternative placements. Both public school programs and residential schools are in danger of disappearing if professionals in the field of vision ignore the threat.

2. Create unified approaches to the resolution of issues in the field of vision for individuals of all ages. It will be necessary for a diverse group of professionals (teachers, O&M specialists, rehabilitation workers, medical-optometric professionals, low vision specialists, technology suppliers, consumers, and parents) to unite, form a structured coalition, and present a single voice on threatening issues. Such unity will probably be most effective at the state level, but it should also be expanded to the national level for some broader issues. It must be done NOW.

3. Collect research data to prove that

    a. generically trained special education teachers are not prepared to instruct students with visual impairments,

b. regular classroom teachers are not prepared to instruct students with visual impairments,

c. students who are visually impaired do not acquire appropriate skills unless they have access to a teacher of the visually impaired, and

d. students who are visually impaired leave the educational system ill-prepared to enter the world of employment if they have not had instruction in disability-specific skills in school.

4. Alert and educate parents about what students with visual impairments may miss if instruction in disability-specific skills is not available. Many parents are unaware that it takes a great deal of specialized training to teach their children what other children learn spontaneously or incidentally. Their voices will carry more weight than almost any other power for change.

5. Plan in-service programs for regular education teachers, to make them aware of the need for a certified teacher of the visually impaired who can provide unique information, instruction, materials, equipment, and philosophical support. Describe the impact of a visual impairment on development, learning, and the acquisition of skills. Present ways of modifying materials and the environment to meet the needs of visually impaired students, but emphasize the individualization of these modifications.

6. Include a strong component of "assessment" in the teacher preparation program for teachers of the visually impaired. This component can be an entire course (which is preferable) or several lectures, but should include a practicum in methods, materials, adaptations, and selected appropriate evaluation procedures.

7. Provide in-service training for school psychologists and/or diagnosticians in assessment techniques for students who are visually impaired. Emphasize the danger of straight visual-to-tactual or visual-to-auditory modifications in test items, the limitations imposed by visual impairment in testing situations, and the need for caution in interpreting test results.

8. Require that a teacher of the visually impaired be a member of the evaluation team at all levels (from referral and screening, to the selection and administration of tests) when the student in question has a visual impairment.

Statement 7

Sophisticated assessments allow the effects of vision to be distinguished from other disabilities present in the multiply handicapped child.

One of the most difficult responsibilities for professionals in the field of visual impairment is the evaluation of individuals who have multiple disabilities. It is especially difficult when one of the disabilities involves the brain, since the brain is the locus of control and monitoring for all other systems in the body. It is nearly impossible to separate the effects of sensory impairments from the effects of brain damage of dysfunction, given the current assessment techniques and technology.

When the effects of individual disabilities cannot be identified in isolation, accurate prescriptions for instruction cannot be made. Programming must allow for interactive functioning between senses and abilities, and such programming is imprecise at best. If it was possible to isolate the effects of various disabilities, more precise instructional strategies could be provided and a more realistic prognosis for learning might be made. As it now stands, neurological dysfunction places a disabled "driver" in the control center, and all other systems in the body are affected. In the case of vision, the major data-collecting sense, impaired function has a reciprocal factor: The control center has insufficient data upon which to base reactions, and reactions become inadequate to control and monitor the collection of data. The interactions multiply to decrease effectiveness. Therefore, the discovery of more sophisticated assessment techniques would be a distinct advancement in evaluating and instructing individuals with multiple handicaps who are also visually impaired.

The participants in this futures study agreed almost unanimously that such a discovery would be a desirable event and that it would probably be made at some point in the future. However, the forces it would take to ensure its occurrence were only moderately stronger than the restraining forces. Among the restrainers were expense, time, lack of expertise by medical specialists, and an insufficient number of researchers who are interested in solving the problem. Moreover, the infinite number of possible combinations of multiple disabilities makes the task even more complicated. It is to the participants' credit that they had the confidence to believe that the future would bring new research, new techniques, and new knowledge.

It is a fact that there has been increased emphasis on brain research in recent years, and scientists are making radical discoveries about brain function. Perhaps professionals in the field of vision should give some priority to reading reports of neurological research, since the implications of this research may extend to other areas, such as vision. New discoveries in neurophysiology may prove to be of help in understanding what visual functioning entails and how it can be enhanced.

Recommendations

1. Create a national office to monitor and disseminate the findings of new brain function. Translate the findings into useful and applicable terms and circulate them among professionals in the field of vision. Be especially aware of research that applies to learning.

2. Encourage doctoral students to explore topics that examine the functional aspects of vision, particularly those that relate to the involvement of and control by the brain. Publish such graduate papers in condensed, readable form, in journals read by professionals in the field of vision.

3. Include a course in neuroanatomy and physiology in teacher preparation programs.

4. Create joint medical-educational teams to evaluate visually impaired students with multiple handicaps. Such children need the cooperative effort of many areas of expertise.

5. Encourage interdisciplinary cooperation in the assessment of visually impaired students with multiple handicaps. Include a neurologist on the team and learn from him or her.

6. Increase the emphasis on assessment techniques, knowledge, and skills at both the preservice and in-service levels.

7. Emphasize the importance of reading medical reports. The teacher of the visually impaired may be able to identify associated etiologies (such as brain tumors or hemorrhages that affect the functioning of the optical nerve or oxygen deprivation and cortical visual impairment) that have an impact on the visual functioning of children with multiple handicaps.

8. Evaluate visually impaired students with multiple handicaps in natural environments, using functional tasks. Emphasize the ability to generalize a skill as part of the criteria for achievement. Collect data on effective instructional techniques, particularly those related to functional vision.

9. Collect data on the effectiveness of visual stimulation with visually impaired students with multiple handicaps. Create controlled conditions and collect consistent data over time.

10. Encourage teachers to share the results of their observations and study of their visually impaired students with multiple handicaps. Publish the results of informal research in professional newsletters and journals.

CLOSING REMARKS

Natalie Barraga opened the symposium by reflecting on the past. She attributed changes to philosophies and practices that center on general attitudes in the field, terminology, organizations and their journals, strategic events, teacher education, research, and literature. She challenged participants to examine how these changes came about and to be open to opportunities to bring about change in the future. We must expand our perspectives through observation and study, take risks by generating creative solutions to problems, and take action when situations demand change. We cannot afford to stand idly by and let the future run over us; too much is at stake. The challenge is to develop and provide the best educational and rehabilitation services for the people we serve. We must consider the entire person, not just isolated facets of his or her academic, social, emotional, health, or employment needs. We must work individually and collectively, we must grow professionally, and we must change systems that are outdated. We must decide on the direction we want to go, chart a course, set sail into sometimes uncharted waters, and believe strongly enough in our goals to persevere through storms and calms alike. There are no precise navigational charts to the future; we are sailing by distant stars. When we fix our gaze on the brightest star, the journey will be worth the effort.

APPENDIX A: FIRST MAILING

<u>COVER LETTER FOR FIRST MAILING</u>

August 23, 1989

Dear Colleague:

The 21st Century is closer than you think! Children who are born this year, 1989, will be voting citizens in the first decade of the 21st Century. Some of these children will be blind or have low vision. What will the world be like for them in the 21st Century? How can we prepare them to function in an age that may be radically different than it is today? What skills will they need, in order to be independent and productive-contributing members of society? Unless we try to anticipate the future, and give some direction to it, we will be <u>subject</u> to it, <u>whatever</u> it will be.

The Program to Prepare Teachers of the Visually Handicapped, at The University of Texas at Austin, is concerned. We believe that, in order to prepare teachers to work more effectively with visually handicapped children, we must understand what those children will need to know when they become citizens of the 21st Century. To accomplish this, we are undertaking a project to forecast the future for visually impaired people. We want to define events that may occur, collect information about those issues, and synthesize this information into forces for change. We want to identify possibilities, and then select those most likely to occur, and which may have greatest impact on visually handicapped children. Most important, we want to know how progress can be managed most effectively, and <u>we need your help.</u>

We have designed a short-term futures project which will collect opinions of knowledgeable people all over the world. It will be a multiple-mailing project (that is, we will ask your opinion several times, over a 3-4 month period). It is important that we collect as many answers as possible, to each and every mailing. You have been selected as a respondent because you have a special interest in the future of visually handicapped persons. Please share your knowledge, feelings, ideas, and opinions with us, by returning all of our surveys. Please complete the enclosed first questionnaire and return it by the due date. (Timing is <u>important,</u> if we are to stay within our established timelines; <u>do</u> observe our response dates.) Instructions for each phase of this project will accompany each mailing.

Help us look at the future with wisdom, foresight, and thoughtful planning. As an educator of visually handicapped children said, at the beginning of the <u>20th</u> Century: "Shall we help it, fight it, or sit still and see if it will run over us?" <u>Their</u> future may have run over them. Help us give <u>direction</u> to the future of <u>today's</u> visually handicapped children.

Thank you for your participation.

Sincerely,

Virginia E. Bishop, Ph.D.   Jane N. Erin, Ph.D.   Anne L. Corn, Ed.D

Note: Please feel free to duplicate these materials and distribute them to as many other people as you wish. We do need to observe our response deadlines in order to stay within the framework of our project timelines, however, so be sure to mention that to others who elect to participate in our study.

INSTRUCTION SHEET & ROLE IDENTIFICATION FOR FIRST MAILING

INSTRUCTIONS

Although we do not need to know your name for the purposes of this project (code numbers are for statistical purposes only), we do need to know your role, for statistical purposes. Please check only one of the following categories - the one that most nearly describes your major role.

_____ Education (either public or private, for B-21 years of age)

_____ Personnel Preparation (college or university level teaching)

_____ Instructional Materials/Resource Center or Library

_____ Rehabilitation (Center, State/Regional Office or Services for Blind Persons over 21 years of age)

_____ Low Vision Center

_____ Parent or relative of a visually handicapped person

_____ Consumer (i.e., a visually handicapped person)

_____ Support agency (e.g., AFB, APH, NAC, NAVH, NSPB, RFB, and federal agencies)

_____ International Professional

_____ Other (please describe)_____

_____

We are asking you to think 25 years into the future - the year 2014.

For each event statement, circle one number to indicate how likely you think it is that the event will actually occur, and one number to indicate how much impact that event would have if it did, in fact, occur.

We are not asking what you would hope will occur, but the likelihood of occurrence, and then how much impact that event would have if it did occur.

Please return this survey **NO LATER THAN SEPTEMBER 15, 1989** in the enclosed envelope or to :

> Dr. Virginia E. Bishop
> Futures Project Coordinator
> The University of Texas at Austin
> EDB 306
> Austin, Texas 78712

FIRST MAILING QUESTIONNAIRE

EVENT	LIKELIHOOD				IMPACT			
	Least Likely		Most Likely		Least Likely		Most Likely	
	1	2	3	4	1	2	3	4
1. An increased understanding of brain and neurological functioning as it relates to sight and seeing, has resulted in improved methods of teaching the visually impaired.	1	2	3	4	1	2	3	4
2. Due to medical and technological advances, the number of visually impaired people have been markedly reduced.	1	2	3	4	1	2	3	4
3. Vision rehabilitation and low vision specialists have emerged as a separate profession from special education.	1	2	3	4	1	2	3	4
4. Environmental simulators, like those used in flight training, have standardized orientation and mobility instruction for those with low vision.	1	2	3	4	1	2	3	4
5. Automatic bank teller machines and other graphic displays have been converted to large print and /or speech output for greater access to the visually impaired.	1	2	3	4	1	2	3	4
6. Reductions in cost and size of low vision aids, along with added versatility have permitted these aids to be "programmed" (computerized) to meet individual needs, pathologies and/or tasks.	1	2	3	4	1	2	3	4
7. Head mounted, miniaturized television cameras, linked electronically to neurological functioning, provide images of the world to the visually impaired.	1	2	3	4	1	2	3	4
8. Child care and early intervention programs for visually impaired children are required to have specially certified teachers.	1	2	3	4	1	2	3	4
9. The increased political power of the aging visually impaired population has resulted in enhanced financial support for health and eye care for visually impaired children.	1	2	3	4	1	2	3	4

EVENT	LIKELIHOOD				IMPACT			
	Least Likely			Most Likely	Least Likely			Most Likely
10. Increased prevalence of low vision among the aging population, has resulted in greater acceptance of individuals with visual impairment.	1	2	3	4	1	2	3	4
11. Socialized health systems exist, and result in prompt referral and appropriate services as standard practice for the visually impaired.	1	2	3	4	1	2	3	4
12. In spite of increasing numbers of minority children with visual impairments, the number of minority professionals in the field has decreased.	1	2	3	4	1	2	3	4
13. Due to increased litigation and bureaucratic constraint, teachers have less contact with families during the educational program planning process.	1	2	3	4	1	2	3	4
14. Improved computer data base management has resulted in interagency (i.e., APH, Library of Congress, RFB, etc.) coordination and more effective tracking and programming for visually impaired children.	1	2	3	4	1	2	3	4
15. Service delivery systems and teaching methodologies for the visually impaired in the year 2014 have not changed appreciably from the standard practices of 1989.	1	2	3	4	1	2	3	4
16. State schools and other institutions for the visually impaired serve only the most severely involved multiply handicapped children.	1	2	3	4	1	2	3	4
17. The knowledge of how children with low vision learn has been greatly expanded; therefore, teachers of the visually handicapped devote more service delivery time to teaching the use of available vision.	1	2	3	4	1	2	3	4
18. Totally blind children are fitted with artificial vision systems; therefore, teachers of the visually impaired utilize competencies appropriate to instructing children with low vision.	1	2	3	4	1	2	3	4
19. Teachers of the visually impaired deliver their services as private practitioners, like psychologists.	1	2	3	4	1	2	3	4

EVENT	LIKELIHOOD				IMPACT			
	Least Likely		Most Likely		Least Likely		Most Likely	
20. Due to the high demand and low supply of teachers for the visually impaired, salary levels are considerably higher.	1	2	3	4	1	2	3	4
21. Low vision and vision rehabilitation specialist services are covered by insurance and health care providers as a part of standard medical practice.	1	2	3	4	1	2	3	4
22. A system of national program evaluation, accreditation and accountability through the National Accreditation Council is implemented fully nationwide.	1	2	3	4	1	2	3	4
23. Computers interpret brain waves, simulating visual experience; functional vision evaluations are no longer required, since professionals can now "view" what a child or adult is seeing.	1	2	3	4	1	2	3	4
24. Disability labels no longer exist relative to education; therefore, individualized assessment of specific disabilities is no longer required.	1	2	3	4	1	2	3	4
25. Sophisticated assessments allow the effects of vision to be distinguished from other disabilities present in the multiply handicapped child.	1	2	3	4	1	2	3	4

APPENDIX B: SECOND MAILING

COVER LETTER FOR SECOND MAILING

September 28, 1989

Dear Colleague,

The response to our first questionnaire was indeed reassuring! Over 200 people were interested in our Futures Project, and sent completed questionnaires. We have analyzed those responses carefully, and are ready to explore the next phase of our Project.

We know what you think is important, and what you feel is likely to occur in the next 25 years. Now we need to know what external forces will be involved in the realization or prevention of the events you told us were likely and that might have impact. We still need your help!

Your opinions and ideas are _very_ important to us. If you shared them with us in the initial phase of this Project-Thank You! If you were not a participant in Part One, you can _still_ help us in _this_ phase. We need as many responses as possible. Please complete the enclosed second questionnaire and return it by the due date, **OCTOBER 20, 1989.** (Timing is _still_ important, if we are to stay within our Project timelines; _do_ observe our response dates.)

Thank you for your continued participation. You are helping to give direction to the future for visually handicapped children.

Sincerely,

Virginia E. Bishop, Ph. D.

Jane N. Erin, Ph.D.

Anne L. Corn, Ed.D.

Note: Please feel free to duplicate these materials and distribute them to as many other people as you wish. We do need to observe our response deadlines in order to stay within the framework of our Project timelines, however, so be sure to mention that to others who elect to participate on our study.

ROLE IDENTIFICATION SHEET FOR SECOND MAILING

INSTRUCTIONS

Please check your role, as you did on the first part of the study. (If you did not participate in the initial survey, you are still invited to complete this phase of the Project.) Please check only one of the following categories -- the one that most nearly describes your <u>major role.</u>

_____ Education (either public or private, for B-21 years of age)

_____ Personnel Preparation (college or university level teaching)

_____ Instructional Materials/Resource Center or Library

_____ Rehabilitation (Center, State/Regional Office or Services for Blind Persons over 21 years of age)

_____ Low Vision Center

_____ Parent or relative of a visually handicapped person

_____ Consumer (i.e., a visually handicapped person)

_____ Support agency (e.g., AFB, APH, NAC, NAVH, NSPB, RFB, and federal agencies)

_____ International Professional

_____ Other (please describe)_____

Please enclose this data sheet with your completed questionnaire. Return both in the enclosed envelope or to :

Dr. Virginia E. Bishop
Futures Project Coordinator
The University of Texas at Austin
EDB 306
Austin, Texas 78712

<u>NO LATER THAN OCTOBER 20, 1989</u>

The results of the first survey indicated a strong likelihood of occurrence, a probable high impact should the event occur, or both, for 12 of the event statements. These are the ones you will be considering further in this part of the Project.

Continue to think about events that might occur 25 years into the future (the year 2014) and do three things for each of the following 12 statements:

1. Decide whether each event statement would be a desirable or an undesirable occurrence, if it really happened, and then check the appropriate box. Do this for each statement.

2. Give at least one facilitating force (something that could cause the event to occur) and at least one restraining force (something that might prevent the event's occurrence. Even if the event is undesirable, the facilitator is still a force that might cause it to occur, and the restrainer is still a force that could prevent it. (It is hoped that you can think of more than two forces for each item!) Do this for every statement.

3. After you have identified the facilitating and restraining forces for each item, assign values to them. (The strongest force would receive the highest value, and the weakest force would receive the lowest value.) It does not matter if the forces are facilitators or restrainers; all forces for each statement should total 10.

Below is a sample item, to illustrate how you might respond to an event statement:

Outcome

EVENT: Service delivery systems and teaching methodologies for the visually impaired in the year 2014 have not changed appreciably from the standard practices of 1989.

[ ] Desirable

[X] Undesirable

Facilitating Forces:	Weight
Shortage of VH teachers	1
High case loads	1
General public attitudes	1
Ineffective child identification and tracking systems	1

Restraining Forces:	
New research put into practice	1
Outreach resource assistance	1
Stronger consumer voice	1
More comprehensive teacher education	3
	10

Remember to do all three steps for each and every event statement. We are anxious to know what you think!

QUESTIONNAIRE TWO: IDENTIFYING FACILITATING AND RESTRAINING FORCES

Example of item from Questionnaire Two:

Event:	Check only one:	Facilitating Forces:	Weight
An increased understanding of brain and neurological functioning as it relates to sight and seeing, has resulted in improved methods of teaching the visually impaired.	[ ] Desirable Outcome [ ] Undesirable Outcome	1. 2. 3. Restraining Forces: 1. 2. 3.	——— ——— ——— ——— ——— ——— 10

The following event statements were also included in the questionnaire from the second phase:

Event: Automatic bank teller machines and other graphic displays have been converted to large print and/or speech output for greater access to the visually impaired.

Event: Reductions in cost and size of low vision aids, along with added versatility have permitted these aids to be "programmed" (computerized) to meet individual needs, pathologies and/or tasks.

Event: Child care and early intervention programs for visually impaired children are required to have specially certified teachers.

Event: Increased prevalence of low vision among the aging population, has resulted in greater acceptance of individuals with visual impairment.

Event: Due to increased litigation and bureaucratic constraint, teachers have less contact with families during the educational program planning process.

Event: Improved computer data base management has resulted in interagency (i.e., APH, Library of Congress, RFB, etc.) coordination and more effective tracking and programming for visually impaired children.

Event: State schools and other institutions for the visually impaired serve only the most severely involved multiply handicapped children.

Event: The knowledge of how children with low vision learn has been greatly expanded; therefore, teachers of the visually handicapped devote more service delivery time to teaching the use of available vision.

Event: Low vision and vision rehabilitation specialist services are covered by insurance and health care providers as part of standard medical practice.

Event: Disability labels no longer exist relative to education; therefore, individualized assessment of specific disabilities is no longer required.

Event: Sophisticated assessments allow the effects of vision to be distinguished from other disabilities present in the multiply handicapped child.

APPENDIX C: FACILITATORS AND RESTRAINERS FOR EVENT STATEMENTS

EVENT STATEMENT

1. An increased understanding of brain and neurological functioning as it relates to sight and seeing, has resulted in improved methods of teaching the visually impaired.

Facilitators

1. Increased research in neurology, ophthalmology, biophysiology, education, and industry (e.g., robots, artificial intelligence)

2. Closer cooperation between medicine and education

3. Advancements in computer technology (e.g., computer imaging)

4. Increased funding for National Eye Institute

5. Cooperative research between medicine and education

6. Translation of research into teaching strategies

7. Fully funded teacher preparation programs

8. Increased interest in functional low vision

9. More comprehensive teacher preparation, including a course in neuroanatomy

10. In-service training to update teacher skills

11. Better ability to diagnose vision problems at birth

12. Liaison personnel to bridge the gap between teachers and researchers

Restrainers

1. Lack of trained researchers

2. Rigidity of medical thinking regarding education

3. Complexity of brain research

4. Difficulties in studying human subjects

5. Lack of interest in research

6. Lack of funding for research

7. Poor communication of research findings (i.e., lag time between research and practice)

8. Lack of cooperation between education and medicine

9. Shortage of VH teachers [teachers of the visually impaired]

10. Teacher training diminishing

11. Fear of/resistance to change

12. Continued concentration on behaviorism

13. Generic education

14. Low visibility because of low prevalence

EVENT STATEMENT

2. Automatic bank teller machines and other graphic displays have been converted to large print and/or speech output for greater access to the visually impaired.

Facilitators

1. Improved technology

2. Pressure from disabled citizens (demand); consumer advocacy

3. Disabilities legislation

4. Businesses willing to install new equipment

5. Consumers willing to learn how to use the new equipment

6. Improved access to businesses (e.g., transportation)

7. Improved economic status of disabled people

8. Increased literacy in the general public

9. Public services (e.g., banks) establishing handicapped outreach

10. More blind people using banks

11. Accessibility becomes a marketing tool

12. Development of private auditory output for devices

Restrainers

1. Insufficient funding for conversions

2. Low incidence need unrecognized by the general public

3. Lack of political concern

4. Lack of consumer demand

5. Greater incidence of opportunity for crime against the disabled

6. Lack of interest by businesses and the business community

7. Voice output a nuisance factor; voice element eliminates privacy

8. Opposition by organizations of the blind

9. Passive public

10. Corporate isolation from the public

EVENT STATEMENT

3. Reductions in cost and size of low vision aids, along with added versatility have permitted these aids to be "programmed" (computerized) to meet individual needs, pathologies and/or tasks.

Facilitators

1. Advances in miniaturization technology

2. Research breakthrough; experimental models available

3. Political support for research and development

4. Cooperative research and shared research findings (e.g., NASA [National Aeronautics and Space Administration], medicine, rehabilitation, education)

5. Greater numbers of low vision people increase awareness and need

6. Consumer demand

7. Increased understanding of visual functioning

8. Insurance coverage for aids

9. Low vision aids appeal to other populations than visually impaired

10. Adequate instruction in the usage of low vision aids

11. Advances in computer programming techniques

12. Growth in the computer industry

13. General acceptance by the public and by users of the value of low vision aids

14. Increased employment of people with low vision, resulting in higher visibility to employers and the general public

15. More informed consumers

Restrainers

1. Lack of funding for research and development

2. Low prevalence/incidence population results in low consumer demand

3. High cost of the aids

4. Fear/lack of acceptance of new aids

5. Lack of cooperation between medicine and rehabilitation

6. Lack of training for professionals

7. Lack of advocacy

8. Lack of training for users

9. Individual needs of visually impaired persons too unique to encourage the development of such aids

10. Lack of documented need for such aids

11. Too task oriented

12. Cosmetically unappealing; inconvenient to carry/use

13. Poor low vision evaluations

14. Pathologies do not reflect functional needs

15. Too "high tech" for most visually impaired people

EVENT STATEMENT

4. Child care and early intervention programs for visually impaired children are required to have specially certified teachers.

Facilitators

1. Parent pressure/advocacy

2. Professional pressure (AER [Association for Education and Rehabilitation of the Blind and Visually Impaired])

3. National emphasis on early intervention

4. Child development research

5. Growing specialization in the vision field

6. Society's move toward individualization

7. Litigation to implement mandates

8. Legislation to require certified VH teachers [teachers of the visually impaired]

9. Greater understanding of the impact of visual impairment on early development

10. Research on the effectiveness of early intervention

11. Significant increase in the number of medically fragile babies with visual impairments (need special attention)

12. Increased salaries for EC-VH [early childhood-visually handicapped] specialists

13. Stipends/monetary encouragement for additional training (e.g., VH [visually handicapped] certification, plus early childhood, or vice versa)

14. Emphasis on preparing the young VH child for later mainstreaming

15. Outcome standards developed for 5 year olds entering kindergarten

16. Specialists better able to help parents deal with implications of disability

17. P.L. 99-457 encourages appropriate and adequate programs

Restrainers

1. Lack of personnel (teachers)

2. Services unavailable in rural areas

3. Resistance to special teachers

4. Lack of teacher preparation programs

5. Lack of early diagnosis of visual impairments

6. Generic special education trend

7. Interdisciplinary jealousy

8. Lack of funding

9. Generic teacher training program

10. Low prevalence of visual impairments

11. Ignoring mandates for specially certified teachers

12. Increased cost of special teachers

13. Insensitivity to the special needs of young visually impaired children

14. Low salaries for special teachers

15. Bickering about certification (who, how, why, where)

16. Cost of securing additional certification

17. Certification requirements vary from state to state

18. VH child generically counted

EVENT STATEMENT

5. Increased prevalence of low vision among the aging population, has resulted in greater acceptance of individuals with visual impairment.

Facilitators

1. Greater media exposure/coverage (TV, radio, magazines, newspapers, movies, etc.) depicting visually impaired persons in a positive manner

2. More active political and social involvement by aging persons with low vision

3. Advocacy for more low vision clinics/services

4. Ophthalmology resident programs develop specialties in geriatric ophthalmology

5. Increased numbers of visually impaired among public officials and entertainers

6. Third-party financial support for vision care

7. General consumer advocacy

8. Elderly visually impaired persons identified sooner, and more adequate services available

9. Aging network well organized

10. Cooperative efforts and knowledge sharing between vision specialists and geriatric specialists

11. Medical advances extending life spans

12. Public use of low vision aids; low vision aids in the workplace

13. Real mainstreaming of low vision adults in the community

Restrainers

1. Elderly not recognized by the general society as a distinct group

2. Awareness may not equal acceptance

3. Acceptance of *aging* persons with visual impairment may not equate with general acceptance of visually impaired persons

4. Aging population less visible (often in segregated residences)

5. Rehabilitation services not provided for elderly, so aging visually impaired persons not seen as independent in public

6. Elderly not viewed as a profitable market

7. Attitudes are slow to change

8. Lack of personnel with specialties in geriatrics (especially in the field of low vision)

9. Economic pressure *lessens* services for the elderly

10. Lack of funding for rehabilitation services for the elderly

11. Persisting stereotypes of "the blind"

12. Resistance by the aging population itself

13. Continued emphasis on "youth"

EVENT STATEMENT

6. Due to increased litigation and bureaucratic constraint, teachers have less contact with families during the educational program planning process.

Facilitators

1. Time constraints because of heavy caseloads

2. Administrators discourage parent involvement

3. Burdensome bureaucracy

4. Paranoia regarding lawsuits

5. Mobile society

6. Conflicting regulations that result in poorly designed services

7. Increased paperwork for teachers

8. As the quality of teachers declines, teachers become implementers instead of planners

9. Family disinterest/apathy

10. Lack of training in how to work with parents

11. Focus on rules/regulations instead of the child

12. Free legal aid for parents

13. Administrative efforts to avoid due process

14. Shortage of teachers

15. More lawyers; more administrators

16. Legal system holding the school more responsible than the family

17. Increased use of courts to resolve problems

18. Mainstreaming not emphasizing the parent's role

19. IEP [Individualized Education Program] process views parent role as token participation; becomes confrontational

20. Teachers intimidated by administrators

21. Liability issues

Restrainers

1. Parent awareness of rights

2. Increase in parent-teacher partnership

3. Complaints are solved before they reach litigation

4. Assertive teachers who are pro-parents

5. Training in consultation methods for teachers

6. Teachers trained to work with parents

7. Relief from paperwork for teachers

8. Extra pay for after-hours consultation with parents

9. Parent leadership training

10. Dedication of teachers

11. Administrators support teachers

12. Voucher system for parents

13. Elimination of frivolous litigation

14. Parental opinions encouraged, respected, and valued

15. Parental decisions honored

EVENT STATEMENT

7. Improved computer data base management has resulted in interagency (i.e., APH [American Printing House for the Blind], Library of Congress, RFB [Recording for the Blind], etc.) coordination and more effective tracking and programming for visually impaired children.

Facilitators

1. Central reporting/data collection agency designated

2. State economic support for the system

3. Decreasing cost of technology

4. Political pressure from agencies

5. More cost-effective for all users; decreased funding makes cooperation essential for survival

6. New software; development of tracking systems

7. Better definitions (e.g., "blind," low vision)

8. Willingness to share information

9. Better communication among agencies

10. Federal support of coordination efforts

11. Technological advances

12. Education/re-education of teachers and other professionals in how to use the system

13. Common desire to eliminate duplication of services

14. Standardizing equipment

15. Improved data collection at entry level

16. Mandatory reporting of visually impaired (or potentially visually impaired) by pediatricians and hospitals

17. Mandatory vision screening of preschoolers (at ages 1, 3, and 5)

Restrainers

1. Increased local control (especially in education)

2. Privacy issues; confidentiality guidelines

3. "Turf protection" by agencies

4. Lack of funding

5. Lack of visionary leadership in agencies

6. Technophobia

7. Cutting of funding in low prevalence areas

8. Adequate translation of data to direct service providers

9. Bureaucracy

10. Lack of communication between agencies

11. Poor data collection at the input level

12. Tracking of numbers rather than people

13. Federal trend toward singular-category counts

14. Lack of field's ability to determine who should maintain the data base

EVENT STATEMENT

8. State schools and other institutions for the visually impaired serve only the most severely involved multiply handicapped children.

Facilitators

1. Narrow interpretation of least restrictive environment

2. Public schools unwilling to serve severely multiply handicapped

3. State school staff unadaptable

4. Funding cuts

5. Deinstitutional movement

6. Expanded public school programs serving a wider range of disabilities

7. Legal impetus for least restrictive environment

8. Higher numbers of multiply handicapped children

9. Generic teacher preparation

10. State school not credible as an educational institution

11. Mainstreaming trend

12. Parent pressure for residential placement

13. Local districts resist serving severely multiply handicapped

14. Concentration of VH teachers [teachers of the visually impaired] in urban areas

15. Lack of cooperation/communication between state schools and public schools

16. Self-perpetuation of institutional bureaucracy

17. Parent has less choice in placement

18. Rigid admission/dismissal procedures discourage short-term placements

19. Need for close/constant supervision for severely multiply handicapped pupils

Restrainers

1. Legal mandates

2. Good state school staffs

3. Short-term services for "normal" or moderately impaired VH [visually handicapped] students available in state schools

4. Recognition of when mainstreaming is appropriate and when it is not

5. Full continuum required

6. Broader interpretation of least restrictive environment

7. Research data comparing mainstreaming and residential school favorably

8. Expanded role of state school to include outreach services, evaluation, resource center

9. Failures in mainstreaming

10. Shortages of teachers in rural areas

11. Focus on short-term placement, with the goal of returning to the home school

12. Lack of funds at the local level

13. Low prevalence of visually handicapped makes hiring VH teacher impractical

14. Openness to most appropriate placement (emphasis on "appropriate")

15. Need for intensified social skill instruction in a secure setting

16. Development of mainstreaming opportunities within the residential school

17. IEPs [Individualized Education Programs] not reflecting the full needs of the child

18. Sense of partnership between state school and public school in educating visually handicapped children

19. Clearer articulation of the role of the residential school

EVENT STATEMENT

9. The knowledge of how children with low vision learn has been greatly expanded; therefore, teachers of the visually handicapped devote more service delivery time to teaching the use of available vision.

Facilitators

1. Recognition that fewer children are totally blind

2. Change of curriculum in teacher preparation, to emphasize low vision

3. Continued research in low vision, especially as it applies to learning

4. Publication/dissemination of relevant research, in-services

5. Increased funding for teacher preparation programs

6. Parent advocacy for improved/appropriate services

7. Research on visual efficiency, to differentiate learnable and generalizable skills

8. Decreased use of "sleep shades" in client training

9. Shortage of VH teachers [teachers of the visually impaired] will require their attention to urgent needs only (e.g., the improvement of visual efficiency)

10. Expanded use of low vision aids and emphasis on *using* any available vision

Restrainers

1. Wide regional variability in the availability of aids and technology

2. Reluctance of teachers and teacher preparation programs to adapt to change

3. Emphasis on "blind" in teacher preparation programs

4. Lack of in-services for VH teachers already in the field

5. Lack of commercially available materials

6. Lack of research on low vision and learning

7. No means of disseminating what is already known

8. No validity in teaching the use of low vision for multiply handicapped individuals

9. Isolation of VH teachers prevents sharing of information

10. Limited research on learning in general

11. Increased student loads

12. Eliminating the notion that encouraging the use of vision is not a negative attitude toward blindness

13. Increased demand for VH teachers to work on more general activities

14. Educational service delivery system inflexible (not enough time to provide adequate/complete services)

15. Pressure to teach all curricular areas

16. Minimal preparation of VH teachers about learning, especially for the low vision child

17. Generic service delivery

18. Lack of qualified personnel

EVENT STATEMENT

10. Low vision and vision rehabilitation specialist services are covered by insurance and health care providers as a part of standard medical practice.

Facilitators

1. Greater acceptance of low vision

2. Federal legislation; recognition and inclusion in Medicare

3. Consumer pressure

4. More low vision clinics

5. Political pressure from agencies

6. Pressure on insurance companies (class action suits, medical advocacy for third-party funding)

7. Insurance reform

8. Certification of low vision specialists; inclusion of teachers as low vision specialists

9. Demonstration of widespread need

10. Coordinated national plan for medical insurance (not necessarily a federal program)

11. More low vision use "on the job"

12. Improved low vision aids

13. Reduced cost of low vision aids

14. Education of physicians about low vision aids

Restrainers

1. Dissonance among and resistance by medical practitioners

2. Insurance coverage dependent on employability

3. Because of low incidence/prevalence of population, lack of political impact

4 Fear of cost, of both services and appliances

5. Lack of referrals by the medical community sends a message that low vision services are not considered important

6. Small field further divided

7. Rising insurance costs

8. Lack of organization for professional input

9. Abundance of nonlicensed providers

10. Abuse in billing by physicians and low vision specialists

11. Low vision services not clearly defined

EVENT STATEMENT

11. Disability labels no longer exist relative to education; therefore, individualized assessment of specific disabilities is no longer required.

Facilitators

1. Generic trend

2. Local option trend

3. Decreased number of special teachers

4. Denial of disabilities on the part of parents

5. Mainstreaming

6. Trend toward regular teachers serving all children

7. Inadequate teacher preparation for assessing children

8. Shortage of special teachers

9. Least restrictive environment misinterpreted/misapplied

10. Federal government trend toward noncategorical "head count"

11. All teachers trained in all exceptionalities

12. Parent pressure against labels

13. Labels counterproductive to the child's self-image

14. Equality concept (in employment as well as education)

15. Disabled rights activism

16. Elimination of VH [visually handicapped] certification

Restrainers

1. Advocacy for individualization

2. Low incidence needs unique

3. Funding structure

4. Fear of lawsuits

5. Improved teacher preparation (especially in assessment)

6. Required practicum in assessment for VH teachers [teachers of the visually impaired]

7. Strict implementation of the laws requiring assessment

8. Joint effort between teachers and parents to maintain individual assessments

9. Recognition that best programs are based on adequate and appropriate preliminary assessment

10. Funding tied to labels

11. VH students recognized as needing special, disability-related assessment

12. Self-interest groups involved in assessment of disabilities

13. Public awareness of special needs

14. Legislative awareness of the need for special teaching methodologies

15. Generic philosophy questioned

EVENT STATEMENT

12. Sophisticated assessments allow the effects of vision to be distinguished from other disabilities present in the multiply handicapped child.

Facilitators

1. Research on assessment; research in VER-type technology

2. Expanded knowledge of etiologies and consequences of visual impairment

3. Awareness of brain/behavior connection

4. Greater knowledge of visual system and component functions

5. Better medical evaluations

6. Links discovered between certain CNS [central nervous system] problems and low vision

7. Simulating machines to simulate visual input to the brain

8. Educational research on learning

9. Better training of teachers and allied personnel to assess

10. Increased population of VH/MH [visually handicapped/multiply handicapped] children provides research subjects and creates a demand for knowledge

11. Improved technology allowing procedures to assess nonverbal children

12. Categorical funding

13. Research to prove effectiveness of low vision training with multiply handicapped children

14. Interagency collaboration

15. Better understanding of multiple disabilities and their interactive effect

16. Evolving of medical/educational diagnosticians

17. Development of reliable and valid instruments or procedures for assessment

18. Outreach training (in-services) to current VH teachers [teachers of the visually impaired], to update their assessment skills

Restrainers

1. Great expense involved

2. Lack of medical expertise in assessment

3. Severity of impairment at the brain level

4. Amount of time required

5. Lack of integrated personnel preparation (all service providers should receive training in assessment; "vision" still too much reserved for VH teachers)

6. Insufficient number of researchers

7. VH component in multiple handicaps not considered important enough

8. Fear of change; maintenance of traditional approaches

9. Less involvement of people from allied disciplines

10. Uniqueness of multiple handicaps (no two alike)

11. Overspecialization, with lessening interdisciplinary cooperation

12. Lack of training in assessment at the teacher preparation level

13. When assessment tools become available, lack of training for teachers in how to use them

APPENDIX D: THIRD MAILING

<u>COVER LETTER FOR THIRD MAILING</u>

November 10, 1989

Dear Colleague:

This is the last phase of the Project, and it may be the most important: this is the **ACTION PLAN.** Your participation is vital!

Your responses to Part Two of the Futures Study were thoughtful and creative. It was probably the most difficult step of the Project, and we appreciate the time you spent in formulating your answers. As a result of your efforts, we were able to select the final five statements for the last phase of our Project. We hope you will respond as promptly and as creatively as you have for the first two parts.

As noted in the previous mailing, you may still complete this last mailing, even if you did not choose to respond to the first two phases of our study.

We will still allow you to duplicate our materials and to circulate them among other professionals, if you so desire. However, we do ask that you (and any others who share these materials) observe the return date, in order to remain within the timelines of our Project.

Please help us with this final request. We value your opinion as a professional, a parent, or a consumer. It is through this sharing of ideas and viewpoints that we can <u>all</u> have the greatest impact on the lives of the visually impaired persons we serve.

Thank you for your participation in this unique and important study.

Sincerely,

Virginia E. Bishop, Ph.D.

Jane N. Erin, Ph.D.

Anne L. Corn, Ed.D.

ROLE IDENTIFICATION SHEET FOR THIRD MAILING

INSTRUCTIONS

Please check your role, as you did on the other parts of the study. (If you did not participate in one or both previous parts of the study, you are still invited to complete this phase of the Project.) Please check <u>only one</u> of the following categories -- the one that most nearly describes your <u>major role.</u>

_____ Education (either public or private, for B-21 years of age)

_____ Personnel Preparation (college or university level teaching)

_____ Instructional Materials/Resource Center or Library

_____ Rehabilitation (Center, State/Regional Office or Services for Blind Persons over 21 years of age)

_____ Low Vision Center

_____ Parent or relative of a visually handicapped person

_____ Consumer (i.e., a visually handicapped person)

_____ Support agency (e.g., AFB, APH, NAC, NAVH, NSPB, RFB, and federal agencies)

_____ International Professional

_____ Other (please describe)_____

Please enclose this data sheet with your completed questionnaire. Return both in the enclosed envelope or to :

> Dr. Virginia E. Bishop
> Futures Project Coordinator
> The University of Texas at Austin
> EDB 306
> Austin, Texas 78712

<u>NO LATER THAN DECEMBER 8, 1989</u>

The following is a sample page from the third questionnaire and a listing of the four additional event statements that were included in the third phase of the project. The facilitating and restraining strategies generated by respondents to the third phase can be obtained from the authors.

Respondent Instructions: Part Two of this Project measured both desirability and forces for the 12 event statements. Of these 12, five statements revealed the need for further exmination of those events. These are the statements you will be thinking about in Part Three of this Project.

Keep in mind that the purpose of this Project is to anticipate the future, and to have some control over its direction. We will be asking you to help us strengthen or weaken the forces that cause an event to occur or that prevent its occurrence. Since each event is different in its desirability and forces, specific instructions will accompany each statement.

The format of each response will be similar. You will be given the event, the facilitating and restraining forces (which were summarized from your responses), and a comment about why the event was chosen for further study. Then, you will be asked to give two strategies--one for helping the event to occur, and one for helping to prevent its occurrence. Strategies should be concrete actions, not philosophical viewpoints. Strategies should be realistic plans for action that could be implemented at some level.

Event:

1. An increased understanding of brain and neurological functioning as it relates to sight and seeing, has resulted in improved methods of teaching the visually impaired.

Comment:

This event was considered to be desirable by ALL respondents, but the restraining forces almost counterbalanced the facilitators in weight. In order to control the outcome of the event, the facilitators need to be strengthened and the restraining forces need to be weakened.

FORCES:

Facilitators

1. Increased research in neurology, ophthalmology, biophysiology, education, and industry (e.g., robots, artificial intelligence)
2. Closer cooperation between medicine and education
3. Advancements in computer technology (e.g., computer imaging)
4. Increased funding for National Eye Institute
5. Cooperative research between medicine and education
6. Translation of research into teaching strategies
7. Fully funded teacher preparation programs
8. Increased interest in functional low vision
9. More comprehensive teacher preparation, including a course in neuroanatomy
10. Inservice training to update teacher skills
11. Better ability to diagnose vision problems at birth
12. Liaison personnel to bridge the gap between teachers and researchers

Restrainers

1. Lack of trained researchers
2. Rigidity of medical thinking regarding education
3. Complexity of brain research
4. Difficulties in studying human subjects
5. Lack of interest in research
6. Lack of funding for research
7. Poor communication of research findings (i.e., lag time between research and practice)
8. Lack of cooperation between education and medicine
9. Shortage of VH teachers
10. Teacher training diminishing
11. Fear of/resistance to change
12. Continued concentration on behaviorism
13. Generic education
14. Low visibility because of low prevalence

Strategy: To assure that this event happens, choose one facilitating force and describe a concrete plan of action to implement it.

Facilitating Force #_____

_____

Strategy: To weaken or nullify one of the problem areas, choose one restraining force and describe a concrete plan of action to implement it.

Restraining Force #_____

Event:

2. Due to increased litigation and bureaucratic constraint, teachers have less contact with families during the educational program planning process.

Comment:

This event was considered to be undesirable by 95% of the respondents, but restraining forces were weak in weight. If the event is to be prevented from happening the facilitators must be weakened and the restrainers strengthened.

Event:

3. Child care and early intervention programs for visually impaired children are required to have specially certified teachers.

Comment:

This event was considered to be desirable by 86% of the respondents, but restricting forces were weighted as too strong. These restraining forces were strong enough to keep the event from occurring. Much greater strength is needed in the facilitating forces, and a great deal of weakening should occur in the restraining forces.

Event:

4. Disability labels no longer exist relative to education; therefore, individualized assessment of specific disabilities is no longer required.

Comment:

This event was considered to be undesirable by 81% of the respondents. The restraining forces should inhibit the event, but they are not strong. Because there may be insufficient strength in the restraining forces, there is danger that the event might occur. If this is to be prevented, the restricting forces will have to be strengthened, and the facilitating forces weakened.

Event:

5.   State schools and other institutions for the visually impaired serve only the most severely involved multiply handicapped children.

Comment:

This was the only event that revealed a split opinion about desirability; 34% of the respondents reported it as desirable, and 59% thought it undesirable. (A few people did not express an opinion.) The weight of the forces strongly supported the event's occurrence, however (i.e., stronger facilitating than restraining forces). Because of this dissonance, a value judgment could not be made. Therefore, responses will understandably reflect the responder's viewpoint.

ABOUT THE EDITORS

Jane N. Erin, Ph.D., is associate professor and coordinator, Programs for the Preparation of Personnel in Visual Disabilities, the University of Texas at Austin, and president, Division on Visual Handicaps, the Council for Exceptional Children. The author and editor of a number of publications dealing with education and visual impairments, including *Dimensions* and *Visual Handicaps and Learning,* she is executive editor of *RE:view* and a recipient of the American Foundation for the Blind's Access Award for Distance Education.

Anne L. Corn, Ed.D., is professor, Department of Special Education, George Peabody College of Vanderbilt University, Nashville, Tennessee, and was formerly professor, Department of Special Education, the University of Texas at Austin. The winner in 1990 of the Distinguished Service Award, Low Vision Section of the American Optometric Association and the American Foundation for the Blind's Access to the Environment Award, she is the author of numerous books, articles, and other publications and a frequent presenter at national and international conferences.

Virginia E. Bishop, Ph.D., is a special education consultant in the area of visual impairments in Austin, Texas. She has been a lecturer at the University of Texas at Austin and, for almost four decades, an educator, researcher, and author of a wide variety of publications in the field in addition to a presenter of numerous workshops on the subject of education and visual impairments.